Manual of Psychosocial Rehabilitation

Edited by

Robert King
Professor of Psychology and Coordinator of Clinical Psychology, Queensland University of Technology, Kelvin Grove, Australia

Chris Lloyd
Principal Research Fellow, Gold Coast Health Service District and Senior Research Fellow, Behavioural Basis of Health, Griffith University, Gold Coast, Australia

Tom Meehan
Associate Professor, Department of Psychiatry, University of Queensland, Australia and Director of Service Evaluation and Research, The Park, Centre for Mental Health

Frank P. Deane
Professor, Illawarra Institute for Mental Health and School of Psychology, University of Wollongong, Wollongong, Australia

David J. Kavanagh
Professor, School of Psychology & Counselling and Institute of Health & Biomedical Innovation, Queensland University of Technology, Kelvin Grove, Australia

Foreword by Gary Bond

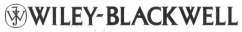

WILEY-BLACKWELL

A John Wiley & Sons, Ltd., Publication

Registered Office
John Wiley & Sons, Ltd, The Atrium, Southern Gate, Chichester, West Sussex, PO19 8SQ, UK

Editorial Offices
9600 Garsington Road, Oxford, OX4 2DQ, UK
The Atrium, Southern Gate, Chichester, West Sussex, PO19 8SQ, UK
111 River Street, Hoboken, NJ 07030-5774, USA

For details of our global editorial offices, for customer services and for information about how to apply for permission to reuse the copyright material in this book please see our website at www.wiley.com/wiley-blackwell

Library of Congress Cataloging-in-Publication Data

Manual of psychosocial rehabilitation / edited by Robert King ... [et al.] ; foreword by Gary Bond.
    p. ; cm.
  Includes bibliographical references and index.
  ISBN 978-1-4443-3397-8 (pbk. : alk. paper)
I. King, Robert, 1949–
  [DNLM: 1. Mental Disorders–rehabilitation. WM 400]
  616.8906–dc23

                       2012008538

A catalogue record for this book is available from the British Library.

Wiley also publishes its books in a variety of electronic formats. Some content that appears in print may not be available in electronic books.

Cover image: iStockphoto/Trout55
Cover design by Andy Meaden

Set in 10/12.5pt Times by SPi Publisher Services, Pondicherry, India
Printed in Singapore by Ho Printing Singapore Pte Ltd

1 2012

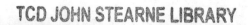

Contents

Foreword

Clinicians in the psychiatric rehabilitation field will welcome this manual for these reasons:

1 *It's realistic.* It addresses common issues in everyday practice, as embodied in "Sam," a fictional yet believable composite client facing a series of life problems. Readers will recognize in Sam the clients they help every day on their recovery journeys. The authors are experienced clinicians who write with conviction and authenticity, as shown in the topics they have chosen and how they write about them. Their choices ring true, consisting of a balance among assessment, counseling, community integration, and self-help. Readers will appreciate the authors' empathy for the challenges facing clinicians.

2 *It's filled with practical tools.* The *Manual* provides scores of user-friendly scales, counseling tips, checklists, and other tools. For example, for assessment tools, the authors give concrete details about ease of administration, scale interpretation, how the scales work in practice, how to obtain copies, and any associated costs. In my experience, clinicians greatly appreciate this tangible help.

3 *It's grounded in empirical research.* Because this manual is a companion book to a handbook explaining the rationale and research foundations for psychiatric rehabilitation practices, readers can be confident that the identified practices have successful track records in helping clients with severe mental illness. And, because the evidence is reviewed in the *Handbook*, the *Manual* can focus exclusively on real-world applications and avoid immersion in the underlying theory and empirical foundations. While the *Manual* can be used as a stand-alone book, the synergy between the two texts invites concurrent reading of relevant material from both sources for deeper understanding.

4 *It presents an integrated approach to psychiatric rehabilitation.* Psychiatric rehabilitation services are fragmented, with practice silos for different psychosocial service areas, such as for illness management, housing, and employment. Comprehensive textbooks mimic usual practice by devoting separate chapters to different service areas, with rare cross-referencing between areas. Clinicians and program managers struggle with coordination and communication between siloed programs. "How do I combine different evidence-base practices? How do they fit together? How do I manage all at once?" Rather than a compendium of practices, the *Manual* aims at a unified narrative by focusing on an individual client. It presents a holistic approach to psychiatric rehabilitation examined through the persona of Sam.

In the Internet Age, you can google anything, but you can't vouch for the credibility of the search results. By contrast, the *Manual* is dependably reliable. It belongs in the clinician's toolbox of frequently-consulted resources.

Gary R. Bond, PhD
Professor of Psychiatry
Dartmouth Psychiatric Research Center
Geisel School of Medicine at Dartmouth
Lebanon, NH, USA

Chapter 1

Introduction

Robert King, Chris Lloyd, Tom Meehan, Frank P. Deane and David J. Kavanagh

Psychosocial rehabilitation (also known as psychiatric rehabilitation) is a term used to refer to a range of non-pharmaceutical interventions designed to help a person recover from severe mental illness.

Severe mental illness is mental illness that is both persistent and has a major impact on life functioning. Schizophrenia is the condition most commonly associated with severe mental illness but it is misleading to associate severity with diagnosis alone. There are many cases of people diagnosed with schizophrenia where the major impact of the illness is brief or where the effect on life functioning is minor. Equally, there are many people with mood and anxiety disorders or with personality disorders whose illness has a major and persistent impact on their life functioning. This book is not concerned with the treatment of a specific diagnostic group but rather with interventions designed to assist people whose mental illness has had a major and persistent impact on life functioning, regardless of diagnosis. It is also designed as a resource and guide for students who are learning how to work effectively with this population. In particular, we see it as an especially valuable resource for the student on placement in settings that provide psychosocial rehabilitation.

Some form of psychosocial rehabilitation is provided in most parts of the world. Sometimes it is provided within long-stay institutional or quasi-institutional settings but typically it is provided by community organisations, which may or may not be affiliated with clinical services. The people providing psychosocial rehabilitation may be health professionals such as nurses, occupational therapists, psychologists and social workers or they may be people without professional training but with skills and attitudes that enable them to assist such people, whether or not they have been trained as health professionals.

Contemporary psychosocial rehabilitation often takes place within a *recovery* framework, which we endorse. The recovery framework emphasises that recovery from mental illness is a process rather than an outcome. Recovery is a personal journey that is about the rediscovery of self in the process of learning to live with an illness rather than being defined by the illness. At an individual level, it is about the development of hope and a vision for the future. At the community level, it is about supporting engagement and

Manual of Psychosocial Rehabilitation, First Edition. Edited by Robert King, Chris Lloyd, Tom Meehan, Frank P. Deane and David J. Kavanagh.
© 2012 Blackwell Publishing Ltd. Published 2012 by Blackwell Publishing Ltd.

participation through provision of opportunity and making connection with the person rather than the illness. The recovery framework informs the way we approach psychosocial rehabilitation. In part, it means that we acknowledge that rehabilitation is only a component of recovery and that it must not seek to over-ride or replace the personal journey. It also means that we approach psychosocial rehabilitation in a spirit of collaboration and partnership with the client. Psychosocial rehabilitation is not something to be imposed on the person and even when, as often is the case, the person is subject to an involuntary treatment order or equivalent, we work with client goals and priorities and negotiate rehabilitation plans.

This book may be seen as a companion to our *Handbook of Psychosocial Rehabilitation* (King *et al.*, 2007). The *Handbook* sets out the principles and evidence base for contemporary practice in psychosocial rehabilitation. This book, which we call the *Manual*, provides the tools and resources to support evidence-based practice. The *Handbook* was well received as a primer in this field of practice but some reviewers noted that while the *Handbook* would assist the reader to work out the best approaches to psychosocial rehabilitation, many readers would still lack the resources to translate principles into practice. We hope that this book will contribute to filling that gap.

Terminology

As with the *Handbook*, we have preferred the term client to patient or consumer. This is based on research indicating that people with severe mental illness identify themselves as patients when in hospital, as clients when receiving community-based services and as consumers when in advocacy roles. We think that the term client both recognises that the service provider has expertise while maintaining an active role for the service recipient as the person seeking and utilising this expertise.

We have also maintained the use of the term rehabilitation practitioner or sometimes just practitioner to refer to the service provider. This recognises that people providing psychosocial rehabilitation come from a wide range of professional and non-professional backgrounds and that what they have in common is that they practise psychosocial rehabilitation.

Organisation of the book

The *Manual* has five main sections.

- Assessment Tools
- Therapeutic Skills and Interventions
- Reconnecting to Community
- Self-Help and Peer Support
- Bringing It All Together

The section on Assessment Tools provides information about standardised instruments that can be used to assist in both initial client assessment and evaluation of client progress.

We have focused on tools that are widely available, have good psychometric properties, are inexpensive or free, have a track record of successful use in psychosocial rehabilitation and require little or no training for use. As well as providing information about specific assessment tools, we provide a guide to when they might be used and information about how to obtain them. In most cases sample items are also provided.

The section on Therapeutic Skills and Interventions contains chapters that provide a 'how to' guide for five interventions. We don't suggest that this is an exhaustive set. However, the interventions chosen have high relevance to psychosocial rehabilitation and a track record for successful application with people who have severe mental illness and do not require extensive training. We do not expect that practitioners will become skilled in provision of these interventions simply by reading this *Manual*. We do, however, think that the *Manual* will provide a good starting point and will enable practitioners to learn from experience. We encourage practitioners to utilise supervision and to access other sources of training in the development of therapeutic skills.

The chapters in Reconnecting to Community set out programmes designed to develop capacity for both independent living and engagement with and participation in the wider community. These include very basic independent living skills, such as money management and cooking, that are often compromised by severe mental illness and more complex social skills that provide the foundation for effective participation in the community. The programmes are typically set out in a week-by-week format for application with groups but there are also tips about adapting the group programmes and tailoring them to individual needs. Many of the activities described will be affected by culture and local environment. We therefore encourage readers to adapt these programmes in accordance with prevailing culture and environment.

The penultimate section of the *Manual* is concerned with peer support, family support and self-help. The rationale for this section is that the evidence suggests that people affected by severe mental illness and those who care for them (especially family members) derive a great deal of benefit from supports and interventions that are substantially outside the psychosocial rehabilitation environment. The rehabilitation practitioner can assist by linking people to such supports and interventions and by providing support to self-help activity. In some circumstances, rehabilitation services may facilitate or sponsor peer and/or family support activities. It is also important for rehabilitation practitioners to be aware of the growing availability of high-quality self-help programmes (especially in the online environment). These can often complement psychosocial rehabilitation interventions provided one to one or in groups. These chapters provide the practitioner with both information and links to resources that will support an effective interface between the rehabilitation environment and the peer support, family support and self-help environments.

The *Manual* ends with two chapters under the heading *Bringing It All Together*. These chapters are concerned with review and evaluation of rehabilitation programmes at individual and service levels. The first of these two chapters focuses on review and redesign of an individual rehabilitation programme. It provides the practitioner with guidance on how to work with a client to identify what has been successful and what remains to be achieved while retaining a positive and strengths-based outlook. The second chapter provides guidance for evaluation of service-based programmes, especially group

programmes. The chapter will assist practitioners to determine whether or not the programmes are achieving the outcomes they were designed to achieve. Together, these two
chapters emphasise that it is not sufficient to provide rehabilitation services. It is important to know that services are achieving expected outcomes both at individual level and
at service level.

Sam

Sam is a young man recovering from severe mental illness. We introduced Sam in the
Handbook and he makes regular appearances throughout this *Manual*. He is of course a
fictional character, being a composite of many people we have worked with in our own
practice experience. We hope that readers will find Sam to be a recognisable person who
embodies many of the challenges and struggles associated with the recovery process. Sam
has been a great help to us as we seek to make psychosocial rehabilitation a living process
rather than an abstraction.

The authors

The authors have professional backgrounds in the fields of mental health nursing, psychology and occupational therapy. Some are primarily in service provision roles and
others work primarily in research and teaching. Most of the authors are based in Australia,
which has a strong international reputation in mental health because of its history of
service planning and service innovation. However, the authors also bring rich international experience as a result of training, working or undertaking research or practice in
various parts of North America and Europe. We have provided some additional information about the contributing editors.

Robert King is a clinical psychologist and professor in the School of Psychology
and Counselling at Queensland University of Technology. He is an editor of the international journal *Administration and Policy in Mental Health and Mental Health
Services Research* and a member of the research advisory committee of the International
Center for Clubhouse Development. Robert worked as a mental health practitioner,
team leader and service manager for 15 years before shifting his focus to teaching and
research. He has strong links and collaborates with mental health researchers in North
America, Europe and Asia. He has published over 100 refereed articles, books and
book chapters in the field of mental health and is a regular contributor to international
conferences.

Frank P. Deane is a clinical psychologist, professor in the School of Psychology and
Director of the Illawarra Institute for Mental Health at the University of Wollongong.
Frank worked as a clinical psychologist in a variety of settings in New Zealand and the
USA before moving to Australia. He is currently the Director of Clinical Psychology
Training at the University of Wollongong. He has published research articles in the area
of help seeking for mental health problems, the role of therapeutic homework in therapy,
medication adherence, recovery from severe mental illness and mental health and drug
and alcohol treatment effectiveness.

David J. Kavanagh holds a research chair in clinical psychology at the Institute of Health and Biomedical Innovation and School of Psychology and Counselling at Queensland University of Technology, and has experience as a clinician and director of a community mental health service, among other roles. He has 28 years of research experience since receiving a PhD from Stanford University and is currently on the editorial boards of three journals, including *Addiction*. He has over 180 publications and leads the award-winning *OnTrack* internet-based treatment team at QUT. David has led or participated in many expert committees on mental health and substance use policy for national and state governments and professional bodies, and has extensive experience in delivering and evaluating training of practitioners in family intervention, co-morbidity and clinical supervision. His applied research has attracted several awards, including a Distinguished Career Award from the Australian Association of Cognitive-Behaviour Therapy in 2011.

Chris Lloyd is an occupational therapist with an extensive background in the area of mental health. She has worked in a variety of settings in Australia and North America with people of different ages and a variety of needs. Chris currently works as the Principal Research Fellow for the Gold Coast Health Service District and is an Adjunct Senior Research Fellow for the Behavioural Basis of Health at Griffith University. Her interests lie in the rehabilitation of people with a mental illness, particularly social inclusion, recovery and vocational rehabilitation. She has published widely, over 150 articles and four books.

Tom Meehan worked as a mental health nurse in Ireland before moving to Australia in 1987. He has worked in a variety of clinical, teaching and research positions and currently holds a joint appointment as Associate Professor with The Park Centre for Mental Health and the School of Medicine at the University of Queensland. Over the past 10 years, Tom has acted as chief investigator for a number of large-scale research and evaluation studies focusing on the rehabilitation of people with psychiatric disability. He has published widely and has delivered papers at professional conferences in Australia and overseas.

Reference

King R, Lloyd C, Meehan T (eds) (2007) *Handbook of Psychosocial Rehabilitation*. Wiley-Blackwell: Oxford.

Part I
Assessment Tools

Chapter 2

Assessment of Symptoms and Cognition

Tom Meehan and David J. Kavanagh

> Sam is a young man who has been diagnosed with schizophrenia. You have been asked to review Sam for a new rehabilitation programme. You are interested in assessing symptom levels and related conditions such as cognitive functioning and substance misuse. It is clear from an interview with Sam that he is experiencing both positive and negative symptoms and he has some difficulty planning activities due to his cognitive impairment. Moreover, he describes difficulty getting off to sleep and feeling 'down' and sad on most days. While Sam claims that his symptoms have deteriorated in recent months, there are no previous assessments of functioning to provide a baseline for comparison. You decide to carry out an overall assessment using a range of measures to assess different aspects of his condition.

Clinical assessment is an integral component of case conceptualisation and treatment planning. While the assessment of symptoms is a major component of any clinical investigation, the assessment of other related conditions such as cognitive impairment and substance misuse should also be considered when determining treatment options for people such as Sam. It is clear that the level of distress experienced due to symptoms will influence the location of treatment (inpatient versus outpatient), the nature and approach to treatment (psychotherapy, medication or both), the level of clinical expertise required to provide the treatment, and the need for other support services such as accommodation, employment or training. Moreover, monitoring symptom levels is useful since a good outcome for many people with severe psychiatric disability is likely to be a reduction in the frequency, duration or severity of symptoms, rather than a complete cure.

Ongoing assessment and monitoring of symptoms and related domains is essential to key decisions such as titrating the degree of support required, providing early intervention to avert relapse, timing new initiatives such as a new job, and negotiating continuance or termination of an intervention. In the absence of adequate monitoring, it can also be difficult to know whether progress is being achieved, especially when it is slow or variable.

In this chapter, we identify a subset of measures that could be used in clinical practice to assess severity of psychotic symptoms, depression, anxiety, substance misuse, and cognitive impairment in people with psychiatric disability.

Manual of Psychosocial Rehabilitation, First Edition. Edited by Robert King, Chris Lloyd, Tom Meehan, Frank P. Deane and David J. Kavanagh.
© 2012 Blackwell Publishing Ltd. Published 2012 by Blackwell Publishing Ltd.

Symptom rating scales

The use of rating scales to assess changes in symptoms increased from the early 1960s, with the need to assess response to emerging psychotropic medications. For example, the Brief Psychiatric Rating Scale (BPRS) was introduced in the early 1960s to assess the effectiveness of chlorpromazine (Overall & Gorham, 1962). At the same time, measures of depression and anxiety, such as those developed by Hamilton, emerged to assess the effectiveness of the new antidepressant medications that were gaining popularity at that time (Hamilton, 1960). While these measures are still widely used, a range of more specific measures has been introduced to assess symptoms in different client groups (adolescents/elderly) and in clinical subgroups such as those with schizophrenia (e.g. the Calgary Depression Scale for Schizophrenia).

Measures described in this chapter

While a broad range of symptom measures currently exists, many are too lengthy, cumbersome and time consuming to be completed routinely by rehabilitation staff. Most of these are more suitable for research and evaluation purposes (e.g. where they may be completed every few months) rather than in clinical practice (where it may be necessary to have measures completed every 1–4 weeks). Therefore, we focus on some of the more clinically useful measures available (Table 2.1). These scales reach a compromise between the burden on the clients and practitioners to complete the measures and the quality of the data they provide. For example, while the BPRS (mentioned above) is a well-recognised measure of symptoms, it is not included here due to the considerable training that is required.

A short description of each measure is provided with an example of its structure. Some of the measures are provided in full (where copyright restrictions allow).

Self-report versus practitioner-rated measures

Approaches to the assessment of symptoms have been developed in two broad formats: (i) self-report measures (completed by the client) and (ii) those administered through interview with a practitioner (practitioner rated). Self-report measures (e.g. Kessler-10) offer some advantages over practitioner-rated measures: they generally take less time to administer and do not require extensive training in their use, making them less expensive to employ. In addition, the information being collected is obtained directly (i.e. without rater interpretation) from the individual being assessed. This is particularly important when collecting client perceptions or subjective experiences (such as in assessments of quality of life and satisfaction). However, self-rating scales do require that clients are able to read and be well enough to understand what is being asked of them. While some self-report measures can validly be administered in an interview format, most have not undergone checking to establish that this is the case, and care needs to be taken to avoid paraphrasing of questions (which may alter their meaning).

Table 2.1   Summary of measures.

Scale	Domains assessed	Structure	Cost
Measures of depressive symptoms			
Calgary Depression Scale for Schizophrenia (CDSS)	Depression in people with schizophrenia	Structured interview (9 items)	No cost
Hamilton Rating Scale for Depression (HAM-D)	Severity of depression	Structured interview (17 items)	No cost
Depression, Anxiety, Stress Scale (DASS)	Depression, anxiety, stress	Self-report (21- or 42-item versions)	No cost
Non-specific measures of psychiatric symptoms			
Behaviour and Symptom Identification Scale (BASIS-32)	Relations to self/others Depression/anxiety Daily living/role functioning Impulsive/addictive behaviour Psychosis	Self-report or practitioner interview (32 items)	Site licence must be purchased
Kessler-10 or Kessler-6	Psychological distress	Self-report (10 or 6 items)	No cost
Clinical Global Impressions (CGI) Scale	Illness severity Improvement Efficacy of medication	Practitioner interview (3 items)	No cost
Measures of cognitive functioning			
Brief Assessment of Cognition in Schizophrenia (BACS)	Verbal memory Working memory Motor speed Semantic fluency Letter fluency Executive function Attention and motor speed	Practitioner administered	Must be purchased
Substance misuse: brief screening measures suitable for repeated use			
DrugCheck Recent Substance Use (RSU)	Quantity/frequency of use in the last 3 months	Self-report/interview (10 substance types)	No cost
Problem List (PL)	Functional impact from most problematic substance in the last 3 months	(12 items)	
Alcohol Use Disorders Identification Test (AUDIT)	Alcohol use and related problems	Self-report (10 items)	No cost
Substance misuse: assessment of consumption			
Timeline followback	Consumption occasions and amounts over recent weeks/months	Self-report/interview	No cost
Opiate Treatment Index (OTI)	Substance use, injecting/ sexual practices, social functioning, crime, health	Self-report in interview (11 substance types, 11 injecting/sexual, 12 social functioning, 4 crime, 50 health)	No cost

People with severe mental illness may not always be able to appraise their own behaviour or performance because of cognitive impairment, or may be unwilling to disclose personal failings, especially if they do not feel it is safe to do so (e.g. if discharge or new opportunities are believed to rest on non-disclosure). The establishment of trust is even more critical than in other contexts and observation or collateral reports may often be necessary to supplement self-reports. While interviews also rely extensively on self-report, they do provide opportunities for observation of behaviour and checking internal consistency of answers.

Assessment of depression

Depression can affect emotions, motor function, thoughts, daily routines such as eating and sleeping, work, behaviour, cognition, libido and overall general functioning. While some scales have attempted to consider all these domains, others have tended to be less inclusive and focus on the main symptoms of depressive illness. More recently, there has been a tendency to develop scales with specific populations in mind (e.g. The Calgary Depression Scale for Schizophrenia).

The Calgary Depression Scale for Schizophrenia

The Calgary Depression Scale for Schizophrenia (CDSS) was specifically designed to assess depression in people with schizophrenia. Unlike some of the other depression measures available, the CDSS includes an assessment of *suicidal thoughts* (Item 8) and *hopelessness* (Item 2). This is an important feature of the CDSS since those with a diagnosis of schizophrenia are at higher risk for suicide (Cadwell & Gottesman, 1990). Moreover, weight changes are not assessed as weight gain/loss can be related to the use of psychotropic medications.

The CDSS contains nine items which are assessed on a four-point response format ('absent' to 'severe'). Eight of the items are completed during a structured interview with the client while the final item (item 9) is based on an overall observation of the entire interview. The domains assessed are outlined in Table 2.2. A total score can be obtained

Table 2.2   Domains included in the Calgary Depression Scale for Schizophrenia.

Item	Domain assessed	Absent	Mild	Moderate	Severe
1	Depressed mood	0	1	2	3
2	Hopelessness	0	1	2	3
3	Self-depreciation	0	1	2	3
4	Guilty ideas of reference	0	1	2	3
5	Pathological guilt	0	1	2	3
6	Morning depression	0	1	2	3
7	Early wakening	0	1	2	3
8	Suicidal thoughts	0	1	2	3
9	Observed depression	0	1	2	3

Box 2.1   Assessment of the Hopelessness domain

- *How do you see the future for yourself?*
- *Can you see any future or has life seemed quite hopeless?*
- *Have you given up or does there still seem some reason for trying?*

0   Absent
1   Mild   Has at times felt hopeless over the past week but still has some degree
                 of hope for the future
2   Moderate   Persistent, moderate sense of hopelessness over the past week
3   Severe   Persisting and distressing sense of hopelessness

---

by summing all item scores to provide a total score of between 0 and 27. A total score of 5 or more is suggestive of depression (in those with schizophrenia).

A glossary is provided for each item to ensure standardisation of the approach followed in the administration of the instrument. The glossary for the *hopelessness* domain is provided in Box 2.1.

Issues for consideration

The CDSS is relatively brief and easy to score, and captures key symptoms of depression in people with schizophrenia. However, it is administered through a structured interview and its developers suggest that users should have at least five practice interviews in the presence of a rater who is experienced in administration of structured instruments before using it alone. Information about the scale and its development can be found in Addington *et al.* (1993), and a copy of the scale and information on its use can be obtained from www.ucalgary.ca/cdss. The CDSS is copyrighted and permission to use it can be obtained by emailing Dr Donald Addington at addingto@ucalgary.ca. It can be used free of cost by students and non-profit organisations.

Hamilton Depression Rating Scale (HDRS)

The Hamilton Depression Rating Scale (HDRS) was developed over 50 years ago and is now one of the most widely used scales for the assessment of depression. The original version included 17 items but a later version included four additional items considered useful in identifying subtypes of depressive illness. However, these four items are not included in the overall rating of depression and the original 17-item version remains more widely used (Bagby *et al.*, 2004).

While the HDRS (also known as the HAM-D) is usually completed following an unstructured interview, guides are now available to assist in having the scale administered in a semi-structured format (see Williams, 1988). Items are scored on a mixture of three-point and five-point scales and summed to provide a total score (range 0–54). It is now widely accepted that total scores of 6 and lower represent an absence of depression, 7–17 mild depression, 18–24 moderate depression and scores above 24 indicate severe depression. Box 2.2 provides an example of the item structure.

Box 2.2   Structure of Hamilton Depression Rating Scale (HDRS)

Instructions: To rate the severity of depression in patients who are already diagnosed as depressed, administer this questionnaire. The higher the score, the more severe the depression. For each item, circle the number next to the correct item (only one response per item).

Item 2: Feelings of guilt
0   Absent
1   Self-reproach, feels he/she has let people down
2   Ideas of guilt or rumination over past errors or sinful deeds
3   Present illness is a punishment. Delusions of guilt
4   Hears accusatory or denunciatory voices and/or experiences threatening visual hallucinations

Item 4: Insomnia (early)
0   No difficulty falling asleep
1   Complains of occasional difficulty falling asleep, i.e. more than half an hour
2   Complains of nightly difficulty falling asleep

Issues for consideration

The HDRS is one of the scales most widely used for the assessment of depression severity. Nonetheless, it has been criticised for not including all the symptoms associated with depression (such as oversleeping, overeating and weight gain) and for inclusion of items related to other domains such as anxiety. Moreover, there are issues with the heterogeneity of rating descriptors for some items; for example, the depressed mood item contains a mixture of affective, behavioural and cognitive features (Bagby *et al.*, 2004).

Notwithstanding these shortcomings, the HDRS is popular in clinical trials and as a measure of depression severity in clinical practice. The scale can be administered in 20–30 minutes, is easy to score (item scores are summed to provide a total score) and there are established 'cut-offs' to indicate levels of depression. However, expertise in the clinical assessment of depression is required, along with training in the use of the scale. There are no restrictions on the use of the scale and copies can be downloaded from http://healthnet.umassmed.edu/mhealth/HAMD.pdf.

Depression, Anxiety, Stress Scale (DASS)

The DASS was developed in Australia (Lovibond, 1998; Lovibond & Lovibond, 1995) and contains 42 items assessing three separate but related constructs: depression, anxiety and stress. A brief version (21 items) is also available, and scores from it correlate highly with the 42-item scale. Responses options focus on the amount of time in the past week that an individual experiences a given problem, such as '*I couldn't seem to experience any positive feeling at all*'. This and other items are rated on a four-point scale ranging from 'Did not apply to me at all' to 'Applied to me very much or most of the time'. The scale's structure is outlined in Box 2.3.

Issues for consideration

The DASS has the advantage of assessing anxiety and stress (in addition to depression) which are frequently found in people with depression. It is completed by the client which

---

Box 2.3   Structure of Depression, Anxiety, Stress Scale (DASS)

Please read each statement and circle a number 0, 1, 2 or 3 which indicates how much the statement applied to you over **the past week**. *There are no right or wrong answers. Do not spend too much time on any statement.*
    The rating scale is as follows:

0   Did not apply to me at all
1   Applied to me to some degree, or some of the time
2   Applied to me to a considerable degree, or a good part of time
3   Applied to me very much, or most of the time

I couldn't seem to experience any positive feeling at all (D)	0	1	2	3
I felt that I was using a lot of nervous energy (A)	0	1	2	3
I found it hard to wind down (S)	0	1	2	3

D, Example of Depression item; A, Example of Anxiety item; S, Example of Stress item.

---

alleviates the need for practitioner training. In the 21-item version, seven items contribute to each of the domains assessed: depression, anxiety and stress. (Each domain in the 42 item version has 14 items.) Item scores in each domain are summed to provide a total score for that domain. The DASS is likely to be more useful in those with less severe problems (i.e. those without psychotic features) as the individual needs to be able to process the statements and provide a response to these. In Australia, the DASS is widely used by general practitioners and other practitioners as a screening tool.

Non-specific measures of psychiatric symptoms

As outlined earlier, a good outcome for many people with mental illness is a reduction in symptom levels. We have selected one client self-report measure to assess distress (Kessler-10) since it requires no training, is brief and easy to score. Moreover, this measure is now included in the suite of measures used to assess client outcomes in Australia. Finally, we have selected the Clinical Global Impressions (CGI) Scale for its brevity and utility in clinical practice.

Kessler 10

The Kessler 10 (K10) was developed to screen for psychological distress in national health interview surveys in the USA (Kessler *et al.*, 2002). Items were primarily derived from existing screening measures on depression, generalized anxiety or positive mood. The K10 (10-question version) provides a global measure of psychological distress based on questions about anxiety and depressive symptoms. All items ask respondents to rate the frequency of the symptom over the past 30 days, using the following options: all of the time (1), most of the time (2), some of the time (3), a little of the time (4), or none of the time (5) (Box 2.4). Scores for each item are summed to provide a total score (range 0–50). Cut-off scores have been developed and suggest that people scoring under 20 are

---

Box 2.4   Structure of Kessler-10

1. During the past 30 days, did you feel tired for no good reason …

| 1. none of the time? | 2. a little of the time? | 3. some of the time? | 4. most of the time? | 5. all of the time? |

---

likely to be well, scores of 20–24 are indicative of mild mental disorder, scores in the range 25–29 represent moderate mental disorder, and scores above 30 represent severe mental disorder. A six-item version of the measure (K6) is also available and the total score derived from this correlates highly with that of the longer version.

Issues for consideration

The K10 is currently used as a client self-rated outcome measure in Australia. Initial feedback indicates that the measure is well accepted by clients and provides useful information to staff for treatment planning purposes. It is also widely used by general practitioners across Australia to screen for anxiety and depressive symptoms. The scale is brief, client rated (no need for staff training) and it is easy to score. However, questions remain about its ability to detect changes in clinical populations (as against its ability to screen for psychological problems). In addition, while the K10 measures distress, it does not cover psychotic symptoms. Notwithstanding this, the K10 is sufficiently brief as to enable additional measures to be used to cover these areas.

Clinical Global Impressions Scale

The Clinical Global Impressions (CGI) Scale (Guy, 1976), is among the brief assessment tools most widely used in clinical trials to provide a brief, global assessment of a patient's functioning prior to and after initiating psychotropic medication. The original version of the CGI had three single-item subscales that asked the treating practitioner to rate (i) illness severity, (ii) improvement and (iii) efficacy of medication, taking into account the patient's clinical condition and severity of side-effects (Guy, 1976). However, the ability of the first two scales to provide an overall assessment of functioning is now recognised. For this reason, only the first two scales are usually employed in clinical practice. The first of these, Severity of Illness (CGI-S), provides a rating of the patient's clinical condition. The practitioner is asked: 'Considering your total clinical experience with this particular population, how mentally ill is the patient at this time?' (rating period is the past 7 days). This question is rated on a seven-point scale ranging from 1=normal to 7=among the most extremely ill patients (see below).

The second scale, the Global Improvement Scale (CGI-I), provides a measure of the patient's improvement or deterioration from a previous baseline assessment using the measure. The practitioner is asked: 'Compared to the patient's condition at admission to the project, how much has the patient changed?'. This question is also rated on a seven-point scale ranging from 1=very much improved to 7=very much worse. Scores on both the CGI-S and the CGI-I are likely to be positively correlated in that change (positive/negative)

Box 2.5   Structure of Clinical Global Impressions (CGI) Scale

1. Severity of illness (CGI-S)
Considering your total clinical experience with this particular population, how mentally ill is the patient at this time?

0 = Not assessed	4 = Moderately ill
1 = Normal, not at all ill	5 = Markedly ill
2 = Borderline mentally ill	6 = Severely ill
3 = Mildly ill	7 = Among the most extremely ill patients

2. Global improvement (CGI-I)
Rate total improvement whether or not, in your judgement, it is due entirely to drug treatment. Compared to his/her condition at admission to the project, how much has the patient changed?

0 = Not assessed	4 = No change
1 = Very much improved	5 = Minimally worse
2 = Much improved	6 = Much worse
3 = Minimally improved	7 = Very much worse

---

on one of the scales tends to be reflected in the other scale. The CGI-S and CGI-I scales are reproduced in Box 2.5.

Issues for consideration

While the CGI was developed as a brief measure of clinical outcome in medication trials, the 'severity' and 'improvement' scales are frequently used (without the Efficacy Index) in routine clinical practice as brief outcome measures. Both scales can be quickly administered by busy practitioners, are easy to score and provide an overall assessment of illness severity and improvement since the commencement of treatment. The CGI is in the public domain and can be used free of cost.

Cognitive functioning measures

It is now clear that people with conditions such as schizophrenia are likely to have some degree of impairment in cognitive functioning (in areas such as working memory, verbal memory and attention). Indeed, these impairments contribute to the severity of disability found in people with schizophrenia (Green, 1996) and tend to predict the outcomes of treatment. The use of cognitive screening is important as it can identify those people who will require additional support and possible cognitive remediation to meet the challenges of community living.

While the Mini-Mental State Examination (MMSE) is one of the better known cognitive assessment scales in the mental health field, it has limited utility in those with schizophrenia. The MMSE was developed for those with organic disorders (such as dementia) who tend to have difficulties with orientation and language. Indeed, people with schizophrenia rated with the MMSE frequently obtain scores within the normal range. Our recommended

---

Box 2.6   Summary of tests included in the Brief Assessment of Cognition in Schizophrenia (BACS)

Verbal memory: Patients are provided with 15 words and then asked to recall them.
Working memory: Patients are presented with a collection of numbers in increasing order. They are then required to repeat the numbers in order, from lowest to highest.
Motor speed: Patients are given 100 tokens and asked to place them in a container as quickly as possible.
Semantic fluency: Patients are given 60 seconds to name as many items as possible one would find in a supermarket.
Letter fluency: Patients are given 60 seconds to name as many words as possible that begin with a given letter such as 'F'.
Executive function: Patients look at two pictures and work out the number of times one would have to move the balls in one picture to make the arrangement in the other.
Attention: Patients are asked to write the numbers 1–9 as matches to symbols on a response sheet.

---

measure is the Brief Assessment of Cognition in Schizophrenia (BACS) since it has demonstrated greater validity and reliability in people with schizophrenia (Keefe *et al.*, 2003).

Brief Assessment of Cognition in Schizophrenia

The BACS has seven separate but related components which assess verbal memory, working memory, motor speed, semantic fluency, letter fluency, executive fluency and attention (Box 2.6).

Issues for consideration

While administration of the BACS requires some training it can be administered by non-psychologists in approximately 35 minutes. The BACS yields a composite score that is comparable to the scores obtained from much longer cognitive assessments in people with schizophrenia (Keefe *et al.*, 2003). The BACS can be purchased from Professor Richard Keefe, Duke University Medical Center, PO Box 3270, Durham, NC 27710, USA, email: Richard.keefe@duke.edu.

Substance misuse measures

Substance abuse is frequently associated with conditions such as schizophrenia and requires careful assessment. Measures for substance misuse are divided into screens for substance-related problems and those to detect changes in substance use or related problems.

Screening measures

Measures to screen for potential substance-related problems need to be sufficiently brief for routine use, and sufficiently sensitive to detect problems reliably in people with mental disorders, while not falsely identifying a large proportion. As the severity of

---

Box 2.7   Structure of the DrugCheck Problem List (PL)

Use this scale after a comprehensive screen of recent substance use.
Ask*: You said you have been recently using (*name substances*). Which of these has caused the most problems or hassles in the last 3 months?* (Use that substance in the questions below)

(If "none": *Which substance would a relative or friend say is causing the most problems or hassles?* If the answer remains "none", omit questions and score zero).

In the last 3 months......

1. Did *(substance)* cause any money problems for you?	0 No	1 A bit	2 A lot
2. Did *(substance)* make you have problems at work, or at school/college/university (use relevant word)?	0 No	1 A bit	2 A lot
3. Did you have housing problems because of *(substance)*?	0 No	1 A bit	2 A lot
4. Were there problems at home or with your family because of *(substance)*?	0 No	1 A bit	2 A lot
5. Did you have any arguments or fights because of *(substance)*?	0 No	1 A bit	2 A lot
6. Has *(substance)* caused any trouble with the law or the police?	0 No	1 A bit	2 A lot
7. Has *(substance)* caused any health problems or injuries?	0 No	1 A bit	2 A lot
8. Have you done anything 'risky' or 'outrageous' after using *(substance)*? (Like driving under the influence, unprotected sex, sharing needles or anything else?)	0 No	1 A bit	2 A lot

Did your use of (substance) in the last 3 months result in you ...

9. Being uninterested in your usual activities?	0 No	1 A bit	2 A lot
10. Feeling depressed?	0 No	1 A bit	2 A lot
11. Being suspicious or distrustful of others?	0 No	1 A bit	2 A lot
12. Having strange thoughts?	0 No	1 A bit	2 A lot

---

mental disorder increases, so does the person's sensitivity to functional impacts from substance use. Anything that substantially affects mood or cognition (e.g. making it harder to judge social situations or detect the difference between illusions or thoughts and hallucinations) can induce psychotic symptoms, and individuals at particularly high risk (or in especially sensitive phases of their illness) are so sensitive to psychoactive substances that a small amount (e.g. of cannabis) on a single occasion can trigger pronounced symptoms. Similarly, people who are barely functioning (e.g. with no disposable income or at risk of losing employment or housing) may have substantial functional impacts from very little substance use. In order to deal with this potential problem, the measures described below are sensitive to less severe forms of substance dependence, in accord with commonly encountered problems in people with psychiatric disorders. The measures were selected for their brevity and their potential to detect change (because of their timeframe and the fact that they offer scaled alternatives rather than relying on presence versus absence).

The DrugCheck Problem List and Recent Substance Use

The Problem List (PL) questions are reproduced in full in Box 2.7. The PL focuses on a substance that the person identifies as producing the greatest current problems for them,

---

Box 2.8   Structure of the DrugCheck Recent Substance Use (RSU)

Items take the form: During the last 3 months have you had any...? If yes: How often have you had that? How much do you usually have?
   Substances/substance types are asked in the order: Tea, coffee or cola drinks? Alcoholic drinks? Cigarettes? Sleeping tablets or sedatives? Painkillers? Marijuana, cannabis or hash? Drugs you sniff, like petrol/glue? Drugs like LSD? Speed, ecstasy, crack or cocaine? Heroin, morphine or methadone? Anything else?
   At least two indicators are used wherever possible (e.g. daily/weekly use, weekly cost), and checks made against collateral or physiological indicators where available. When indicators are in conflict, the person is asked to assist the assessor in determining the best estimate of use from all available data.

---

and is normally preceded by a review of the quantity and frequency of all recent substance using the Recent Substance Use (RSU) drug check (see Box 2.8).

The PL's 12 items form a single factor and cover functional and symptomatic impacts of substance use. A total score of 2 or more on the scale detects 97% of people with psychosis and a current *Diagnostic and Statistical Manual* (DSM)-IV substance-related diagnosis, and falsely identifies only 16% (Kavanagh *et al.*, 2011). All the items contribute to the prediction, although the first eight items are almost as good at detecting substance-related problems as the full set of 12.

Issues for consideration

A significant strength of the PL is its ability to feed into a subsequent motivational interview, providing data on areas seen as 'downsides' of current use of a specific substance. However, current psychometric data on the PL are based on samples of inpatients with psychosis, and further research needs to be undertaken in people with other mental disorders before we can be confident in its performance and in the cut-offs to screen positive in those contexts. A significant strength is the inclusiveness of its items, e.g. any risky or outrageous behaviour, any problems with the law or the police, which are likely to capture the wide range of potential problems this group commonly has.

The focus of the PL on a single substance is both a strength and limitation: a strength, in that it encourages the person to consider one substance that they may wish to change, and a limitation, in that effects of a single substance can be difficult to disentangle from those of others the person is concurrently using. In addition, they may decide to address another substance as their initial target, so a later readministration of the PL may be insensitive to the changes they have made. To detect the overall impact of substance use, the PL can be readministered for each type of substance the person is currently using, but then it becomes a much longer instrument and is less compatible with use by time-poor practitioners. The PL could in principle be applied to substance use in general but data supporting that application are not as yet available.

The RSU attempts to increase accuracy by using triangulation of consumption estimates from multiple indicators (e.g. amount per day or week, amount purchased, reports of other informants, physiological measures), although it remains restricted by its focus on

---

Box 2.9   Structure of the Alcohol Use Disorders Identification Test (AUDIT)

1. **How often do you have a drink containing alcohol?**
   Never (0)   Monthly or less (1)   2–4 times a month (2)   2–3 times a week (3)
   4 or more times a week (4)

2. **How many drinks do you typically have on a typical day when you are drinking?**
   1 or 2   3 or 4   5 or 6   7 to 9   10 or more

3. **How often do you have six or more drinks on an occasion?**
   Never (0)   Less than monthly (1)   Monthly (2)   Weekly (3)   Daily or almost daily (4)

These first three items constitute the AUDIT-C. Estimates of numbers of drinks are assisted by reference to figures displaying the size of 'standard' drinks (in Australia and UK, drinks with 10 g ethanol; in USA drinks with 12 g ethanol).

Items 3–8 (frequency of six or more drinks, loss of control, failure to do what was normally expected, morning drinking, guilt or remorse, memory loss) are scored 0 (never), 1(less than monthly), 2 (monthly), 3 (weekly), 4 (daily or almost daily).

Items 9–10 (injuries, others showing concern or suggesting reduction in drinking) are scored 0 (no), 2 (yes, but not in the last 6 months) or 4 (yes, in the last 6 months).

Screening criteria may differ across countries and are often lower for women, but some data on people with serious mental disorders suggest that a total score score ≥8 indicates presence of an alcohol use disorder.

'typical' consumption. The PL's simple grading of severity ('a bit'/'a lot') makes it easier to use than if greater articulation were attempted; while it may reduce its ability to detect small changes in functional impact, it may also avoid a false sense of accuracy.

Alcohol Use Disorders Identification Test

The Alcohol Use Disorders Identification Test (AUDIT) (Saunders *et al*., 1993) is a 10-item scale covering alcohol consumption and problems in the last 6–12 months (Box 2.9). It has been validated for use in a wide variety of contexts, including people with serious mental disorders. In Kavanagh *et al*. (2011), a cut-off of at least 8 on the Australian version of the scale (which slightly changes item 2, to detect whether respondents are using quantities above the Australian guidelines of the time) detected 96% of inpatients with psychosis who also had alcohol abuse or dependence, and incorrectly identified 20% as having the co-occurring disorder. In Maisto *et al*. (2000), these figures using the standard AUDIT were a little poorer, at 90% and 30% respectively.

Issues for consideration

The first three items, which focus on consumption, carry much of the predictive variance of the AUDIT and are sometimes used alone as the AUDIT-C. Since they focus on current consumption, they can be used as a brief indicator of change, although greater accuracy in estimating consumption will be gained from recording the actual frequency of typical drinking and of binge drinking, and obtaining an estimate of the number of drinks typically consumed. Accuracy further increases if assessments move beyond 'typical' consumption to typical consumption on particular days of the week or fortnight (if drinking shows predictable weekly or bi-weekly variations) or, better still, if occasions of recent drinking are reconstructed using the Opiate Treatment Index or Timeline Followback (reviewed below).

Items 4–10 use the timeframe of the past year and in some cases focus on potentially infrequent events (e.g. injuries) or indices of physical dependence (e.g. morning drinking). They therefore have less utility as an indicator of change over short periods of time.

Estimates of consumption – measures

Consumption and related risk behaviours typically change before improvements in functioning or reductions in physical dependence can reliably be detected. Measures of consumption that give increased accuracy also tend to incur somewhat greater time or cost than the more simple estimates of typical recent use provided by the RSU and AUDIT.

Timeline Followback

The Timeline Followback involves using a calendar format to record daily events or activities that the individual recalls occurring over the past 2 weeks to 3 months. These events or activities may be personal or family routines or one-off events, holidays or festivals, or memorable news items. The events are used to cue recall of purchase and daily consumption of substances over the period. In people with serious mental disorders, we usually focus on the last 2–4 weeks, recording all substance use, and then ask whether that period was typical of the previous 3 months. If there were times when consumption was higher or lower, we attempt to determine the duration of those periods and the extent of consumption at those times. This approach allows an estimation of current and recent consumption levels of all substance types, while keeping the required time for assessment relatively short. No special materials are needed for the assessment, beyond a blank calendar with space to record events and substance use.

Issues for consideration

The Timeline Followback has shown high levels of agreement with daily alcohol self-monitoring and biochemical measures. It has the advantages of being able to be used retrospectively, without having to rely on patients remembering to monitor their behaviour, is not subject to loss of monitoring forms, and can extend reporting beyond the limits imposed on biochemical measures by metabolism of the substance. However, it relies on relatively intact memory and sustained attention, and can require some time to complete if multiple substances are used frequently. In cases where one or more substances are used infrequently, some flexibility with the reporting period is required (asking about the last 2–3 occasions of use over the period since the previous assessment rather than focusing solely on a shorter timeframe). In common with other self-report measures, its accuracy also requires that trust has been developed, and in particular, that disclosure of substance use will not result in negative outcomes.

Box 2.10   Structure of the Opiate Treatment Index (OTI)

Items about drug use take the form of this example.
Now I'm going to ask you some questions about heroin (smack, hammer, horse, scag).

1. On what day did you last use heroin?
2. How many hits/smokes/snorts did you have on that day?
3. On which day before that did you use heroin?
4. And how many hits/smokes did you have on that day?
5. And when was the day before that?

Recent consumption is indexed by the total consumption across the last two occasions, divided by the sum of the days between the last three occasions of use.
  Social functioning items include housing stability, employment in the last 6 months, conflict with relatives, partners or friends, number of close friends, satisfaction with social support, frequency of contact with friends, number known for more than 6 months, time with other users, number of friends who are users.

A sample item is:
How often in the last 6 months have you had conflict with your relatives?

Very often	4
Often	3
Sometimes	2
Rarely	1
Never	0
N/A	

Opiate Treatment Index

The Opiate Treatment Index (OTI) is a self-report instrument that is administered by interview (Box 2.10). After biographical and treatment details, it asks about the most recent 3 days of substance use: in order, heroin, other opiates, alcohol by type, cannabis, amphetamines, cocaine, tranquillisers, barbiturates, hallucinogens, inhalants and tobacco. The timing and amounts of the substance use allow calculations of average consumption of each substance type per day (totalling the last two amounts and dividing by the sum of the days between the last three occasions). It then asks about injecting practices, sexual behaviour, social functioning, crime and health problems.

Issues for consideration

A focus on the last three consumption days reduces reliance on memory and allows for estimations of both frequently used substances and more infrequent consumption. However, it relies on those occasions being representative, and if there is systematic variation over time (e.g. more use on the weekends or more use after pension day), the estimate may not be accurate. It therefore needs to be combined with questions about representativeness and, if necessary, additional instances may be required. While the omission of related events shortens the assessment, it also loses the benefit of those events cueing more accurate recall. As the title of the measure implies, it emphasises issues around heroin and other illegal substance use; beginning with heroin (as against caffeine in the DrugCheck) may inhibit free admission of use in cases where the person is worried about reporting illegal or injected substance use, and may alienate people who are only using legal substances. Along the same lines, drink or drug driving, the most common illegal behaviour of substance users, is omitted. On the other hand, the breadth of questions on health, needle use, risky sexual practices and social issues is a significant strength.

Use of the measures in practice

During an interview with Sam, you notice that his mood appears to be flat and he complains that the illness has '*destroyed my life and there is nothing to live for any more*'. You assess for depression using the CDSS). His total scale score is 9 which indicates possible depression (cut-off for depression is a score of 5 or more).

You consider using the BASIS-32 to assess symptoms but feel that Sam may not be able to cope with such a detailed assessment. You decide to use the CGI scale to obtain a global measure of severity. Sam obtains a score of 5 (out of a possible score of 7) on the 'severity' subscale and a score of 3 (out of a possible score of 7) on the improvement subscale. This suggests that the severity of his illness remains high and his level of improvement is low.

During the interview with Sam, he mentions that he has been drinking far more than he usually does. You consider each of the reviewed assessment scales/methods described above and decide to use a combination of the approaches as this may prove superior. After establishing rapport with Sam, a DrugCheck RSU is initially used to determine which substances had been used since the last assessment. Alcohol emerges as the substance causing most impact on Sam's functioning. You continue the assessment of alcohol use using the DrugCheck Problem List to assess the functional and symptomatic impact of alcohol use. Sam receives a score of 7 which indicates that he has significant problems with his alcohol use.

A more extensive Timeline Followback could then be administered where there appeared to be variability over time (e.g. on different days of the week) or when greater accuracy was needed (e.g. to detect small changes in consumption). Further checks on the representativeness of the selected period would then be undertaken (e.g. asking about the timing of abstinence periods, using other events to anchor recall). In cases where there may be reasons to doubt self-report (e.g. rewards are provided if the person is abstinent or rapport is uncertain), some form of biochemical assay of urine, saliva or blood could be employed.

Summary

In this chapter we have reviewed a small number of measures that could be considered for the assessment of symptoms, cognitive impairment and substance misuse. These measures are readily available, brief to complete, easy to score and have acceptable psychometric properties. Given these features, the measures described are more likely to be acceptable to the busy rehabilitation practitioner. While the measures described may prove useful for clinical and evaluation purposes, none of the scales described is designed to replace a thorough clinical assessment. The selection of the most appropriate instrument will need careful appraisal of the clients to be assessed (age, cultural background, ability to read and write, cognitive impairment, stage of illness), the amount of data required, the training of raters, the time and costs involved (self-report versus client interview), and the availability of raters with sufficient clinical experience.

References

Addington D, Addington J, Maticka-Tyndale E (1993) Assessing depression in schizophrenia: the Calgary Depression Scale. *British Journal of Psychiatry* **163**(Suppl 22), 39–44.

Bagby R, Ryder A, Schuller D, Marshall M (2004) The Hamilton Depression Rating Scale: has the gold standard become a lead weight? *American Journal of Psychiatry* **161**, 2163–77.

Cadwell C, Gottesman I (1990) Schizophrenics kill themselves too: a review of risk factors for suicide. *Schizophrenia Bulletin* **16**, 571–89.

Green M (1996) What are the functional consequences of neurocognitive deficits in schizophrenia? *American Journal of Psychiatry* **153**, 321–30.

Guy W (1976) Clinical Global Impressions (CGI). In: *Assessment Manual for Psychopharmacology*, revised edition. US Department of Health, Education, and Welfare: Washington, DC.

Hamilton M (1960) A rating scale for depression. *Journal of Neurology, Neurosurgery and Psychiatry* **23**, 56–62.

Kavanagh DJ, Trembath M, Shockley N *et al.* (2011) The DrugCheck Problem List: a new screen for substance use disorders in people with psychosis. *Addictive Behaviors*. Available at: http://dx.doi.org/10.1016/j.addbeh.2011.05.004.

Keefe R, Goldberg T, Harvey P (2003) The Brief Assessment of Cognition in Schizophrenia: reliability, sensitivity, and comparison with a standard neurocognitive battery. *Schizophrenia Research* **68**, 283–97.

Kessler R, Andrews G, Colpe L *et al.* (2002) Short screening scales to monitor population prevalence and trends in non-specific psychological distress. *Psychological Medicine* **32**, 959–76.

Lovibond P (1998) Long-term stability of depression, anxiety, and stress syndromes. *Journal of Abnormal Psychology* **107**, 520–6.

Lovibond S, Lovibond P (1995) *Manual for the Depression Anxiety Stress Scales (DASS)*, 2nd edn. Psychology Foundation: Sydney.

Maisto SA, Carey MP, Carey KB, Gordon CM, Gleason JR (2000) Use of AUDIT and the DAST-10 to identify alcohol and drug use disorders among adults with severe and persistent mental illness. *Psychological Assessment* **12**, 186–92.

Overall J, Gorham D (1962) The Brief Psychiatric Rating Scale. *Psychological Reports* **10**, 799–812.

Saunders JB, Aasland G, Babor TF, DE LA Fuente JR, Grant, M (1993) Development of the Alcohol Use Disorders Identification Test (AUDIT): WHO collaborative project on early detection of persons with harmful alcohol consumption: II. *Addiction* **88**, 791–804.

Williams J (1988) A structured interview guide for the Hamilton Depression Rating Scale. *Archives of General Psychiatry* **45**, 742–7.

Chapter 3

Assessment of Functioning and Disability

Tom Meehan and Chris Lloyd

In a recent interview with Sam, it became clear that he had problems with everyday functioning, particularly in the areas of self-care and social interaction. Sam was wearing crumpled clothes that looked dirty and smelled as if they had not been washed for some time. He said he was attending church regularly but enquiries revealed he was not interacting with anyone else at church. You have concerns that Sam will be unable to address these impairments without significant input from the rehabilitation team. You also wonder what other difficulties he is having with his everyday functioning. As his rehabilitation worker, you decide to carry out an in-depth assessment of his functioning to identify areas requiring attention and to provide accurate information for his rehabilitation plan. You also want to get reliable baseline information so that you can evaluate the success of interventions put in place to assist him.

Introduction

While the positive symptoms of psychotic conditions such as schizophrenia tend to plateau and even cease following the active phase of the illness, deficits in functioning (i.e. disability) can continue to accumulate. Indeed, limitations in functioning can represent a significant component of illness burden (Bellack *et al.*, 2006). It is now clear that conditions such as schizophrenia have a pervasive impact across a wide range of life domains. Initial assessment and ongoing monitoring of deficits in functioning using standardised measures should be a major focus of rehabilitation workers. In this chapter we build on the work outlined in the previous chapter (which addressed the assessment of symptoms) and focus on the assessment of functioning.

Functioning is a broad and complex construct that encompasses a number of related domains such as role, relationships, leisure, self-care, and physical and psychological health (Mueser & Gingerich, 2006). In addition, there are a number of related factors that can affect functioning such as insight and the impact of medication side-effects. Since there is currently no single scale available to assess all of these constructs, we have identified a range of measures that could be considered for monitoring and evaluation purposes (Table 3.1).

Manual of Psychosocial Rehabilitation, First Edition. Edited by Robert King, Chris Lloyd, Tom Meehan, Frank P. Deane and David J. Kavanagh.
© 2012 Blackwell Publishing Ltd. Published 2012 by Blackwell Publishing Ltd.

Table 3.1   Summary of functioning and disability measures.

Measure	Domains assessed	Administration	Cost
Assessment of impairment			
Health of the Nation Outcome Scales (HoNOS)	Behaviour Impairment Symptoms Social functioning	12 items/scales Completed based on client interview, client observation and information from carers, etc.	No cost
Assessment of functioning			
Life Skills Profile (LSP-16)	Withdrawal Self-care Compliance Antisocial behaviour	16 items Completed based on client observation and information from carers and others	No cost
Multidimensional Scale of Independent Functioning (MSIF)	Work Education Residential Each domain is rated on 3 aspects: role, support and performance	3 domains (rated on 3 aspects) Semi-structured interview with client	No cost
Multonmah Community Ability Scale (MCAS)	Functioning Adjustment to living Social competence Behavioural problems	17 items Practitioner version Client version (self-report)	Copyright Fee for use
Independent Living Skills Survey (ILSS)	Personal hygiene Appearance and clothing Care of personal possessions Food preparation Care of health and safety Money management Transportation Leisure and recreation Job seeking Job maintenance Eating behaviours Social interactions	103 items practitioner version 51 items self-report version	Copyright Fee for use
Assessment of insight			
Birchwood Insight Scale (BSI)	Insight into illness	8 items Completed by client	No cost, no permission needed
Assessment of side-effects			
Liverpool University Neuroleptic Side-Effect Rating Scale (LUNSERS)	Extrapyramidal side-effects Autonomic side-effects Psychic side-effects Anticholinergic side-effects Allergic reactions Prolactin-related side-effects Miscellaneous side-effects	51 items Completed by client	No cost

Assessment of impairment

Health of the Nation Outcome Scales

The Health of the Nation Outcome Scales (HoNOS) were developed in the UK by Wing and associates as a measure of illness severity (Wing *et al.*, 1996) (Box 3.1). The HoNOS comprise 12 separate but related scales, which address problems in four areas.

- *Behavioural problems* (aggression, self-harm and substance use)
- *Impairment* (cognitive and physical)
- *Symptomatic problems* (hallucinations/delusions, depression and other symptoms)
- *Social problems* (relationships, daily living, housing and work)

Each scale is rated from 0 ('no problem') to 4 ('severe to very severe problem'). The total score for all 12 scales ranges from 0 to 48 where higher scores represent greater overall severity. The rating period is usually the previous 2 weeks.

The HoNOS has been validated in Canada (Kisely *et al.*, 2006), the UK (Bebbington *et al.*, 1999) and Australia (Trauer *et al.*, 1999). Indeed, the HoNOS is now included in the suite of measures used in Australia to monitor outcomes for clients in receipt of mental health services.

Issues for consideration

The HoNOS is completed by a mental health professional following an interview with the individual being rated. In most cases, the client will be able to provide sufficient information to complete the HoNOS. However, in situations where the client is unwilling or unable to participate in the assessment, the rater will need access to information from a relative or carer. For example, Scale 1 asks for information about aggressive incidents in the past 2 weeks. Clients may be unwilling to discuss this and additional information from a carer may be required.

While the instrument appears to be relatively straightforward, its completion can be demanding. Clinical judgement is required and the rater will also need to consult a glossary as each scale is being completed. Face-to-face training using the programme developed by

---

Box 3.1   Example of Health of the Nation Outcome Scales – item 3, problems with drinking or drug taking

Do not include aggressive/destructive behaviour due to alcohol or drug use, rated in Item 1. Do not include physical illness or disability due to alcohol or drug use, rated in item 5.

Glossary for item 3

0 No problem of this kind during the period rated
1 Some overindulgence but within social limits
2 Loss of control of drinking or drug taking, but not seriously addicted
3 Marked craving or dependence on alcohol or drugs with frequent loss of control, risk taking under the influence (e.g. drunk driving)
4 Incapacitated by alcohol/drug problems

Source: Royal College of Psychiatrists, London.

the College of Psychiatrists is recommended. In addition, copyright in the scale is owned by the Royal College of Psychiatrists and permission to use the scale must be obtained from the College. The contact is:

The Training Program Manager
Royal College of Psychiatrists
17 Belgrave Square
London, SW1X 8PG
email: egeorge@rcpsych.ac.uk

Those interested in the HoNOS may wish to visit http://www.rcpsych.ac.uk/training/honos.aspx for a more in-depth discussion of the measure and training requirements.

Assessment of daily functioning

Disability associated with disorders such as schizophrenia can have a major impact on one's ability to perform basic self-care activities. Understanding the challenges that individuals have in meeting the basic necessities of life (cooking, cleaning, shopping, managing finances, meeting healthcare needs, etc.) will form a key component of any rehabilitation assessment. A wide range of measures is now available to assess these areas of functioning and a selection of those more commonly used in in the rehabilitation field, are discussed below. The focus is on those applicable to those with severe disability. Some are self-rated by the client whereas others are completed by the rehabilitation worker.

The Life Skills Profile

The Life Skills Profile (LSP) was developed in Australia as a multidimensional measure of functioning and disability in people with schizophrenia (Rosen *et al.*, 1989). However, the LSP is now applied more broadly since many of the 'skills' assessed are also relevant in other psychotic and organic conditions. The LSP is rated by a practitioner using observable behaviours rather than clinical assessment or interview.

Three versions of the LSP have emerged: the LSP-39 (original version), the LSP-20 and LSP-16. The original 39-item version was found to be rather lengthy for routine use by practitioners and this led to the development of the two briefer versions (Trauer *et al.*, 1995). The LSP-16 was developed as a measure of outcome for the Mental Health Classification and Service Costs Project, a case-mix initiative implemented in Australia in 1996 (see www.mnhocc.org). The 16-item version is included in the suite of measures currently used to monitor client outcomes in Australian mental health services (Meehan *et al.*, 2006).

The 16 items are summed to yield four subscales (withdrawal, self-care, compliance and antisocial behaviour) and a total scale score. Items are scored 0–3 where '0' represents low levels of dysfunction and '3' represents high levels of dysfunction (Box 3.2).

Issues for consideration

The Life Skills Profile is a useful measure for the assessment of rehabilitation outcomes since aspects of functioning ('life skills') rather than symptoms are assessed. Indeed,

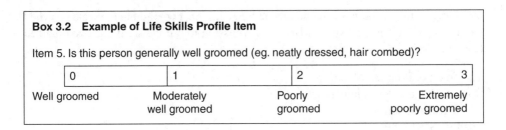

the domains assessed via the LSP (withdrawal, self-care, compliance and antisocial behaviour) will often be the focus of rehabilitation efforts. Unlike some of the other measures reviewed, the LSP can be used to assess those attending both inpatient and outpatient rehabilitation programmes. The period covered by the scale is the previous 3 months and the rater needs to be familiar with the functioning of the client over that period. The measure can be used by clinical and non-clinical raters and no specific training is required as the measure has well-described anchor points. While there are currently three versions of the scale in use, these are scored differently and, when comparing findings with published reports in the literature, it is important to check that the version you are using is similar to that used in the published report.

Copies of the LSP-39, LSP-20 and LSP-16 and other relevant information concerning the structure and scoring of the different versions of the scale can be downloaded from http://www.blackdoginstitute.org.au/research/tools/index.cfm.

Multidimensional Scale of Independent Functioning

The Multidimensional Scale of Independent Functioning (MSIF) is a relatively new instrument for rating functional disability in psychiatric outpatients (Jaeger et al., 2003). The scale captures a 1-month time period and is completed by a mental health professional following a semi-structured interview with the individual being rated. The interview guide is available from the authors of the scale (see details below).

The interview provides for a thorough analysis of the person's day-to-day activities in each of the three domains:

- work (e.g. competitive, supported, dependent care, volunteer)
- education (e.g. college, vocational or certificate school, rehabilitation training programme)
- residential (e.g. where the person is living, what responsibilities the person has).

If the individual is working and in training, both work and training are rated. However, education is rated only if the individual is enrolled in training/education. Similarly, work is rated if the client is in some form of work.

Each of the three domains (work, education and residential) are coded according to a detailed set of anchors to provide an assessment of (i) role, (ii) support and (iii) performance for each of the three domains. For example, when the 'work' domain is assessed, the rater would consider the job title, the type of work carried out, when and at what pace tasks are performed, the level of supervision required, the level of assistance required, and the overall performance standard of the work. Each dimension is rated along a seven-point Likert scale (1 = normal functioning to 7 = total disability). Global ratings can be obtained for each domain (work, education, residential) and for each dimension (role, support and performance). Finally, a global rating (total scale score) can be obtained for overall functioning.

Issues for consideration

While this is a relatively complex measure, it provides a more comprehensive assessment of work, education and living arrangements than most of the other instruments reviewed. The provision of extensive detail for each anchor point reduces the need for rater interpretation/judgement and increases inter-rater agreement. No specific training is required to use the measure. The collection of information concerning support and performance improves the ability of the scale to differentiate between higher and lower functioning individuals. This feature of the MSIF improves its capacity to identify change following clinical interventions and makes it particularly useful in the evaluation of rehabilitation programmes that focus on improving work, training and residential capacity. Follow-up assessments can be conducted via telephone and provide information on changes in role position, level of support required, and performance level achieved. The scale was developed for outpatients and captures a 1-month timeframe (this can be adapted to monitor a longer period). A detailed description of the MSIF is provided in the article published in *Schizophrenia Bulletin* by Jaeger *et al.* (2007).

The interview schedule and copies of the MSIF can be obtained without cost from:

Professor Judith Jaeger
Department of Psychiatry and Behavioural Sciences
Zucker Hillside Hospital
75–59 263rd Street
Glen Oaks, NY 11004
email: jaeger.ju@comcast.net

Multonmah Community Ability Scale

The Multonmah Community Ability Scale (MCAS) (Barker *et al.*, 1994) was designed to assess the level of functioning in clients with more severe disability living in community settings. The scale contains 17 practitioner-rated items that can be collapsed into four subscales or domains of functioning.

- *Interference in Functioning* (five items focusing on physical health, mental health, intellectual health)
- *Adjustment to Living* (three items dealing with daily living skills and money management)
- *Social Competence* (five items that assess social interest and skills)
- *Behaviour Problems* (four items that assess participation in treatment, substance use and acting-out behaviours)

The rating period for items in the first three domains is the past 3 months while the fourth domain assesses functioning in the past 12 months. All items are scored on a five-point

---

Box 3.3   Example of Multnomah Community Ability Scale item

1. How impaired is the client by his/her physical health status? Note: Impairment may be
   from chronic health problems and/or frequency and severity of acute illnesses.

1. Extreme health impairment   ☐
2. Marked health impairment   ☐
3. Moderate health impairment   ☐
4. Slight health impairment   ☐
5. No health impairment   ☐

---

scale and item scores are summed to provide a domain score and total scale score
(Box 3.3). Barker and colleagues (1994) suggest that total scale scores of 17–47 indicate
severe disability, 48–62 represent medium disability, and 63–85 indicate little or no
disability. The measure has high predictive validity – individuals with lower scores
were more likely to be hospitalised at some time in the future (Hampton & Chafetz,
2002). The measure has adequate inter-rater and test-retest reliability (Trauer, 2001).

Issues for consideration

The MCAS is a useful measure for the assessment of functioning in clients with severe
disability living in the community (rather than in inpatient settings). While the subscale
scores may be useful from a clinical perspective, the total score is likely to be more reliable (Corbiere et al., 2002). The measure, which takes about 10 minutes to complete,
needs to be administered by a practitioner or other provider familiar with the client. In
addition, information from all available sources, including family, carers and rehabilitation staff, needs to be considered when rating the measure. Training in the use of the
measure is recommended. A self-report version of the measure (i.e. the MCAS-SR) was
developed in 2002 by O'Malia and colleagues. These authors found the MCAS-SR to be
reliable and acceptable to clients.

A copy of the scale can be downloaded from www.ct.gov/dmhas/LIB/dmhas/MRO/
multnomhah.pdf. However, both versions of the MCAS are copyrighted. In addition to
the payment of a fee to use the measures, a one-off site licence is required. Information
concerning this, and a training video, can be obtained from Network Ventures Inc. at
www.multonamahscales.com.

Independent Living Skills Survey

The Independent Living Skills Survey (ILSS) is a comprehensive, objective, performance-
focused, easy-to-administer measure of the basic functional living skills of individuals
with severe mental illness (Wallace et al., 2000). This measure has two versions, one for
staff and other informants (ILSS-I) and another that can be completed by clients/self-report
(ILSS-SR). The staff version contains 103 items, which assess performance in 12 areas
of basic community living skills (these are listed in Table 3.1 above). Staff/informants
indicate how frequently an individual has performed each skill within the past month

Table 3.2 Example of Independent Living Skills Survey (informant version).

How often did the person perform each behaviour in the past 30 days?	Always	Usually	Often	Sometimes	Never	No
Food preparation and storage						
Prepared simple foods such as sandwiches, cold cereal, etc. that did not require cooking	☐	☐	☐	☐	☐	☐
Discarded spoiled foods (without prompting)	☐	☐	☐	☐	☐	☐

on a five-point scale (never, sometimes, often, usually, and always) (Table 3.2). Scores are then summed and averaged per functional area (items rated as 'no opportunity' are ignored in the scoring process). A higher score indicates better functioning. The ILSS-I can be conveniently administered in person, by phone or by mail, because completion requires only a brief oral or written explanation of the response scale. The measure takes around 20 minutes to administer.

The ILSS-SR was developed to provide a simplified version of the ILSS-I. This version has 51 items and assesses functioning in 10 domains. In addition, the response format was simplified to 'yes', 'no' and 'does not apply' to make it easier for individuals with severe mental illness to complete the measure. Both versions of the measure have acceptable reliability and validity (Wallace *et al.*, 2000).

Issues for consideration

The informant version of the measure (i.e. the ILSS-I) can be applied by anyone familiar with the patient. It is easy to score and interpret and could be used to monitor rehabilitation interventions as it has demonstrated ability to detect change. Copies of both versions of the measure are available in the article published in *Schizophrenia Bulletin* by Wallace *et al.* (2000). However, both versions of the ILLS are copyrighted and a small fee is payable. Information concerning this, and a training video, can be obtained from http://www.psychrehab.com/assessment/assessment_ilss.html.

Other measures of functioning

The measures of functioning discussed above represent only a small sample of the many measures that are available. In Table 3.3 we have identified three other measures that could be considered when assessing functioning in individuals with serious mental illness.

Assessment of insight

Lack of insight is frequently found in clients with psychotic conditions. Although the concept is poorly understood, it is thought to have an impact on compliance with treatment, aggressive behaviour, self-harm and overall prognosis (Birchwood *et al.*, 1994;

Table 3.3   Additional measures of functioning.

Measure	Brief description
University of San Diego (UCSD) Performance-based Skills Assessment (UPSA)	The UPSA is a performance-based measure of everyday functioning in clients living in the community (Patterson *et al.*, 2001). It was designed to assess skills in five areas: household chores, communication, finance, transportation and planning recreational activities. The UPSA involves role-play tasks similar in complexity to situations that a community-dwelling person is likely to encounter. A summary UPSA score is calculated by summing these five scores. The total time for completing the UPSA is approximately 30 minutes. A brief version of the measure (i.e. UPSA-B) has been developed and this takes 10–15 minutes to complete (Mausbach *et al.*, 2007)
Camberwell Assessment of Need Short Appraisal Schedule (CANSAS)	The Camberwell Assessment of Need Short Appraisal Schedule (CANSAS) is a structured interview in which staff, client and carer views of need can be recorded separately (Andresen *et al.*, 2000). It was designed specifically to inform clinical practice and to serve as a service evaluation tool. Each of the 22 domains is rated as no serious problem (no need), or no problem or a moderate problem owing to help given (met need), or a serious problem, irrespective of help given (unmet need)
St Louis Inventory of Community Living Skills (SLICLS)	The St Louis Inventory of Community Living Skills (SLICLS) was developed as a relatively brief level of functioning measure, with a focus on discrete community living skills (Evenson & Boyd, 1993). The scale was designed to be useful in measuring the level of specific skills needed for community or group home residence. This measure can be completed in 2 or 3 minutes by someone familiar with the client. Each item is rated on a seven-point scale from few or no skills to self-sufficient, very adequate. Validity and reliability scores for the SLICLS are adequate (Fitz & Evenson, 1995)

McEvoy, 1998). Insight is said to be present if the individual has some awareness of his/her emotional state and absent if the individual vigorously denies that he/she is ill (World Health Organization, 1973). Although the quantity of measures available to assess insight is limited, available measures tend to focus on similar concerns: acceptance of illness, the need for treatment and willingness to take medications. The insight scale developed by Birchwood is included here since it is brief, has good psychometric properties and can be completed through self-report by the client.

Birchwood Insight Scale

The Birchwood Insight Scale (IS) was developed in the UK by Max Birchwood and colleagues (Birchwood *et al.*, 1994). The scale comprise eight statements (four positively worded and four negatively worded) which are rated on a three-point scale (agree, disagree, unsure) (Table 3.4).

Table 3.4   Birchwood Insight Scale – complete measure.

Instructions: Please read the following statements carefully and then circle the number that best applies to you	Agree	Disagree	Unsure
1. Some of the symptoms were made by my mind	2	0	1
2. I am mentally well	0	2	1
3. I do not need medication	0	2	1
4. My stay in hospital was necessary	2	0	1
5. The doctor is right in prescribing medication for me	2	0	1
6. I do not need to be seen by a doctor or psychiatrist	0	2	1
7. If someone said that I had a nervous or mental illness then they would be right	2	0	1
8. None of the unusual things I experience are due to an illness	0	2	1

The eight items can be collapsed into three domains of insight.

- Awareness of symptoms (items 1 + 8), maximum score = 4
- Awareness of illness (items 2 + 7), maximum score = 4
- Need for treatment (items 3 + 4 + 5 + 6). Divide by 2 to provide subscale total. Maximum score = 4.

A total scale score is derived by summing the three subscale scores (range 0–12), with a higher score indicating higher levels of insight. The IS has moderate internal reliability (Cronbach's alpha = 0.75) and high test-retest reliability (0.90) (Birchwood *et al.*, 1994).

Issues for consideration

The IS provides a brief self-report measure of insight in individuals with mental illness. The scale has been widely used in the assessment of insight in research and clinical samples. The scale has been found to be reliable, valid and sensitive to change (Birchwood *et al.*, 1994). While the scale was developed for inpatients, it can also be used in community populations. Item 4 ('My stay in hospital was necessary') is not included in the version provided to those living in the community.

There is no cost associated with the use of the scale and permission to use the scale is not required. The scale can be reprinted from Table 3.4. Additional information can be obtained from Professor Max Birchwood at: m.j.birchwood.20@bham.ac.uk.

Assessment of side-effects

Antipsychotic medications continue to play a significant role in the treatment of serious mental health conditions. Modern medications, although not curative, have altered the course of disorders such as schizophrenia by reducing positive symptoms, improving clinical stability and reducing relapse rates (Hogarty & Ulrich, 1998). However, despite advances in the development of these medications, many patients continue to experience unpleasant side-effects from their use (Meehan *et al.*, 2011). These effects frequently impact on their ability to carry out daily tasks and may lead to poor compliance with medication regimes (Awad & Voruganti, 2004). A growing literature suggests that mental health workers have difficulty recognising the side-effects of psychotropic medications (Coombs *et al.*, 2003; Morrison *et al.*, 2000). The use of assessment tools specifically designed to assess medication side-effects is likely to assist practitioners in this process. The major benefit of identifying adverse side-effects is that it opens the way to investigating changes in medication type and/or dose so as to minimise adverse effects of treatment and secondary effects such as non-compliance.

A growing number of measures are currently available for the assessment of side-effects. These range from global measures such as the Liverpool University Neuroleptic Side-Effect Rating Scale (LUNSERS) to more specific measures that focus on extrapyramidal side-effects. For example, the Simpson-Angus Scale (SAS) is a useful measure of rigidity and tremor (Simpson & Angus, 1970) while the Barnes Akathisia Rating Scale (BARS) provides an assessment of restlessness and the distress associated with medications (Barnes, 1989). Given that the 'motor' side-effects associated with the newer atypical antipsychotics appear to be less distressing (Hagan & Jones, 2005), information derived from the LUNSERS may prove more useful in clinical practice since it provides assessment of a broad range of side-effects.

Liverpool University Neuroleptic Side-Effect Rating Scale

The LUNSERS was developed in the UK by Day and colleagues (1995) to monitor medication-induced side-effects. In contrast to most of the other scales designed to assess side-effects, the LUNSERS was designed to be completed by clients (rather than clinical staff). The measure includes a total of 51 side-effects of which 41 are recognised side-effects and 10 are false side-effects (known as 'red herrings'). The red herring side-effects (such as chilblains, hair loss, runny nose, etc.) are used to identify individuals who may be over-rating their side-effects. All 51 side-effects are rated on a five-point scale ranging from 'not at all' to 'very much' (Table 3.5).

The 41 recognised side-effects can be collapsed into seven domains.

- Extrapyramidal – parkinsonion type side-effects
- Autonomic – includes uncontrollable side-effects
- Psychic – relates to the functioning of mind and emotion
- Anticholinergic – side-effects affecting the choline system
- Allergic reactions – such as skin rashes
- Prolactin – related to hormones such as prolactin
- Miscellaneous – side-effects without a clear category

Table 3.5   Example of LUNSERS item/structure and scoring.

Please indicate how much you have experienced each of the following symptoms in the past month	Not at all (0)	Very little (1)	A little (2)	Quite a lot (3)	Very much (4)
Difficulty staying awake during the day	☐	☐	☐	☐	☐

Issues for consideration

The LUNSERS is longer than most side-effect measures but it does enable assessment of a broad range of adverse effects. In addition, the measure is completed by the client (rather than the practitioner) and since many side-effects are subjective (e.g. psychic side-effects), it is likely that a self-completed measure would provide a more valid rating. Due to the length of the measure, clients with more severe impairment may need support to complete it. While the measure can be scored by hand, a computer program is available to assist with data management and calculation of scores for each of the seven domains (described above).

Sam's functional assessment

You commence Sam's assessment by inviting his mother to complete the Life Skills Profile (LSP-16) which provides an indication of the level of disability he has in caring for himself. Sam obtained a total score of 18 (out of a possible score of 48) which indicates he has moderate levels of disability (lower score indicates lower levels of disability). Further information on scores for Australian samples can be obtained from www.mhnocc.org. Examination of the subscale scores showed that Sam has serious deficits in his self-care and strategies to address this should be a focus in his rehabilitation plan.

During discussions with Sam you note that he appears to have a poor understanding of his illness. You ask Sam to complete the Birchwood Insight Scale to assess his understanding of his condition. Sam obtained a score of 4 out of a possible score of 12 on the scale which indicates that he has little or no insight into his illness (lower score indicates poorer insight). Indeed, he obtained a score of 0 on the 'awareness of illness' subscale which highlights his lack of insight on illness awareness. People with mental illness may be willing to acknowledge experiencing stress or other difficulties and accepting treatment for these but low insight scores should alert the practitioner to the need for ongoing education to improve insight.

While undertaking this assessment, you notice that Sam is restless and he has difficulty concentrating on the questions being posed. During your next meeting with Sam, you ask him to complete the LUNSERS. His overall LUNSERS score was 76 (out of a possible total scale score of 156). The most severe problems are noted in the psychic subscale, in which Sam obtained a score of 31 out of a possible subscale score of 40 (higher scores represent more severe problems). Items receiving high scores included difficulty with concentrating, remembering things and tiredness. These could be part of the negative symptom profile of his mental illness but it is possible that they are, in part, side-effects of his medication. It is well worth alerting Sam's treating doctor to this possibility. If symptoms persist despite an optimal medication regime, Sam might be a candidate for cognitive remediation (see Chapter 9).

Feedback to clients, families and carers and others in the treating team

As you have now collected a considerable amount of information, this will prove useful in providing a baseline for future assessments. You should also provide feedback to the various people who need to know, starting, in this case, with Sam himself. The provision of feedback to clients is an important aspect of treatment evaluation. Allen and colleagues (2003) found that clients who received feedback following assessments had higher satisfaction with the assessment process than those who received no feedback.

The provision of feedback needs to be carried out sensibly so as not to overload the client and/or family and carers with too much detail. Feedback also must be provided sensitively so as not to be discouraging. The focus of feedback should be on the client's strengths rather than his/her deficits (Gamble & Brennan, 2006). The amount of detail provided to individuals will depend on their ability to comprehend the information being provided. For example, some clients may appreciate a simple discussion of what was found while others may value summary graphs/scores that compare the present results to those of previous assessments.

Feedback to colleagues is particularly important when it has potential to affect the wider treatment plan. Such feedback should highlight possible implications for other areas of treatment.

Summary

While a plethora of measures has been developed to assess 'functioning', no single measure is currently available to assess the broad range of domains included under the umbrella of 'functioning'. Many existing measures have problems with scope, validity, reliability, floor/ceiling effects and applicability (Bellack et al., 2006). Moreover, many measures of functioning are lengthy and cumbersome to score and as such, have limited utility when applied in the clinical setting.

Notwithstanding these concerns, standardised measures yield systematic information which might be overlooked in routine clinical practice. They also provide a quantitative basis for evaluation of progress in treatment.

Decisions around the most appropriate measure will depend on a number of factors such as the frequency of assessment ('one-off' versus routine), the resources available to administer the measures, and the level of disability in the target group (this may dictate whether practitioner-rated or client-rated measures are to be used). In addition, clear guidelines and data management systems need to be established to facilitate the reporting/use of the data derived from assessments. While staff, clients and their carers frequently spend considerable time completing assessment measures, many of these are rarely discussed with clients or considered in service planning and evaluation activities (Meehan et al., 2006).

References

Allen A, Montgomery M, Tubman J, Frazer L, Escovar L (2003) The effects of assessment feedback on rapport building and self-enhancement processes. *Journal of Mental Health Counselling* **25**, 165–81.

Andresen R, Caputi P, Oades LG (2000) Interrater reliability of the Camberwell Assessment of Need Short Appraisal Schedule. *Australian and New Zealand Journal of Psychiatry* **34**, 856–61.

Awad G, Voruganti L (2004) New antipsychotics, compliance, quality of life, and subjective tolerability. Are patients better off? *Canadian Journal of Psychiatry* **49**, 297–301.

Barker S, Barron N, McFarland B, Bigelow D (1994) A community ability scale for chronically mentally ill clients: Part I. Reliability and validity. *Community Mental Health Journal* **30**, 363–83.

Barnes T (1989) A rating scale for drug–induced akathisia. *British Journal of Psychiatry* **154**, 672–6.

Bebbington P, Brugha T, Hill T, Marsden L, Window S (1999) Validation of the Health of the Nation Outcome Scales. *British Journal of Psychiatry* **174**, 389–94.

Bellack A, Green M, Cook *et al.* (2006) Assessment of community functioning in people with schizophrenia and other severe mental illness: a White Paper based on an NIMH-sponsored workshop. *Schizophrenia Bulletin* **33**, 805–22.

Birchwood M, Smith J, Drury V, Healy J, Macmillian F, Slade M (1994) A self-report Insight Scale for psychosis: reliability, validity and sensitivity to change. *Acta Psychiatrica Scandinavica* **89**, 62–7.

Coombs T, Deane F, Lambert G, Griffiths R (2003) What influences patient medication adherence? Mental health nurse perspectives' and a need for education and training. *International Journal of Mental Health Nursing* **12**, 148–52.

Corbiere M, Crocker A, Lesage B, Latimer E, Ricard N, Mercier C (2002) Factor structure of the Multnomah Community Ability Scale. *Journal of Nervous and Mental Disease* **190**, 399–406.

Day JC, Wood G, Dewey M Bentall R (1995) A self-rating scale for measuring neuroleptic side effects. Validation in a group of schizophrenic. *British Journal of Psychiatry* **166**, 650–3.

Evenson RC, Boyd MA (1993) The St Louis Inventory of Community Living Skills. *Psychosocial Rehabilitation Journal* **17**, 93–7.

Fitz D, Evenson RC (1995) A validity study of the St Louis Inventory of Community Living Skills. *Community Mental Health Journal* **31**, 369–77.

Gamble C, Brennan G (2006) Assessments: a rationale for choosing and using. In: Gamble C, Brennan G (eds) *Working With Serious Mental Illness: A Manual for Clinical Practice*. Elsevier: London, pp.111–31.

Hagan J, Jones D (2005) Predicting drug efficacy in schizophrenia. *Schizophrenia Bulletin* **31**, 830–53.

Hampton M, Chafetz L (2002) Factors associated with residential placement in an assertive community treatment program. *Issues in Mental Health Nursing* **23**, 677–89.

Hogarty G, Ulrich R (1998) The limitations of antipsychotic medication on schizophrenia relapse and adjustment and the contributions of psychosocial treatment. *Journal of Psychiatric Research* **32**, 243–50.

Jaeger J, Berns S, Czobor P (2003) The Multidimensional Scale of Independent Functioning: a new instrument for measuring functional disability in psychiatric populations. *Schizophrenia Bulletin* **29**, 153–67.

Kisely S, Campbell LA, Crossman D, Gleich S, Campbell J (2007) Are the Health of the Nation Outcome Scales a valid and practical instrument to measure outcomes in North America? A three-site evaluation across Nova Scotia. *Community Mental Health Journal* **43**, 91–107.

Mausbach T, Harvey P, Goldman S, Jeste D, Patterson T (2007) Development of a brief scale of everyday functioning in persons with serious mental illness. *Schizophrenia Bulletin* **33**, 1364–72.

McEvoy J (1998) The relationship between insight in psychosis and compliance with medications. In: Amador X, David A (eds) *Insight and Psychosis*. Oxford University Press: New York, pp.289–306.

Meehan T, Coombs S, Hatzipertou L, Catchpoole R (2006) Practitioner reactions to the introduction of routine outcome measurement in mental health. *Journal of Psychiatric Mental Health Nursing* **13**, 581–7.

Meehan T, Stedman T, Wallace J (2011) Managing the side effects of antipsychotic medications: Consumer perceptions. Australasian Psychiatry 19, 74–77.

Morrison P, Meehan T, Gaskill D, Lunney P, Collings P (2000) Enhancing case managers' skills in the assessment and management of antipsychotic medication side-effects. *Australian and New Zealand Journal of Psychiatry* **34**, 814–21.

Mueser K, Gingerich S (2006) *The Complete Family Guide to Schizophrenia: Helping Your Loved One Get the Most Out of Life*. Guilford Press: New York.

Patterson TL, Goldman S, McKibbin CL, Hughs T, Jeste DV (2001) UCSD Performance-based skills assessment: development of a new measure of everyday functioning for severely mentally ill adults. *Schizophrenia Bulletin* **27**, 235–45.

Rosen A, Hadzi-Pavlovic D, Parker G (1989) The Life Skills Profile: a measure assessing function and disability. *Schizophrenia Bulletin* **15**, 325–37.

Simpson G, Angus J (1970) A rating scale for extrapyramedial side effects. *Acta Psychiatrica Scandinavica* **212**(Suppl), 11–19.

Trauer T (2001) Sympton severity and personal functioning among patients with schizophrenia discharged from long-term hospital care to the community. *Community Mental Health Journal* **37**, 145–55.

Trauer T, Duckmanton RA, Chui E (1995) The Life Skills Profile: a study of its psychometric properties. *Australian and New Zealand Journal of Psychiatry* **29**, 492–9.

Trauer T, Callaly T, Hantz P, Little J, Shields R, Smith J (1999) Health of the Nation Outcome Scales. *British Journal of Psychiatry* **174**, 380–8.

Wallace C, Liberman R, Tauber R, Wallace J (2000) The Independent Living Skills Survey. *Schizophrenia Bulletin* **26**, 631–58.

Wing JL, Curtis RH, Beevor AS (1996) *HoNOS: Health of the Nation Outcome Scales. Report on Research and Development, July 1993–Dec 1995*. College Research Unit, Royal College of Psychiatrists: London.

World Health Organization (1973) *Report of the International Pilot Study of Schizophrenia*, vol 1. World Health Organization: Geneva.

Chapter 4

Assessment of Recovery, Empowerment and Strengths

Tom Meehan and Frank P. Deane

> It is clear that Sam feels demoralised by his illness. It is not that he is depressed but rather that he does not have any vision of the kind of life he wants to lead or any confidence in his ability to develop a worthwhile life despite his illness. You feel that engaging him in rehabilitation can assist him to develop greater hope and self-efficacy and you are looking for ways in which you can check in with Sam to see if he is making progress in these areas.

The previous two chapters in this book provide pointers for rehabilitation workers when assessing illness components such as symptoms, impairment and functioning. While assessment of these domains provides important information for planning and evaluation purposes, the focus tends to be on the 'clinical' presentation of the individual and the identification of symptoms and functional deficits that need to be 'fixed'. Clients have been critical of traditional mental health services for paying undue attention to these clinical outcomes and insufficient regard to the subjective, personal and 'internal' knowledge of the individual (Glover, 2005).

Over the past 20 years, individuals with mental illness and client advocacy groups have been promoting broader concepts such as recovery, strengths and empowerment. Indeed, these concepts have now become the guiding vision for mental health service delivery (Deegan, 1996; Rapp & Goscha, 2006; Segal *et al.*, 1995). Emerging evidence suggests that a greater focus on these domains is likely to improve the clinical outcomes for people with psychiatric disability (Corrigan, 2006; Hasson-Ohayon *et al.*, 2007; Rapp & Goscha, 2006).

It is becoming increasingly important for practitioners working in the rehabilitation field to include some assessment of these domains in their work with clients. However, unlike the broad range of measures available to assess symptoms and functional impairment, there is a paucity of standardised measures available to assess domains such as empowerment and strengths. From an extensive review of the literature, we have identified two measures that could be used to assess individual recovery, one measure of empowerment and two measures commonly used to assess strengths. These five measures were selected based on their availability, ease of use, brevity and sound psychometric properties (Table 4.1).

Manual of Psychosocial Rehabilitation, First Edition. Edited by Robert King, Chris Lloyd, Tom Meehan, Frank P. Deane and David J. Kavanagh.

Table 4.1   Recovery, empowerment and strengths measures.

Scale	Domains assessed	Structure	Cost
Recovery measures			
Recovery Assessment Scale (RAS)	Personal confidence and hope Willingness to ask for help Goal and success orientation Reliance on others No domination by symptoms	Self-report Original version (41 scaled items). Short version (24 scaled items). Both versions assess the same five domains	No cost
Illness Management and Recovery Scales (IMR)	Personal goals Social supports Substance use Functioning Medication adherence Coping skills Participation in meaningful activities	Self-report Client and practitioner versions (each version contains 15 items)	No cost
Empowerment measures			
Making Decisions Empowerment Scale	Self-esteem and self-efficacy Power and powerlessness Community activism Optimism and control over future Righteous anger	28 scaled items	No cost (small licensing fee if used in conjunction with other measures from Ohio site)
Strengths measures			
Strengths Assessment Worksheet	Daily living situation Financial/insurance Vocation/education Social support, health Leisure/recreation Spirituality/culture	Semi-structured interview	No cost (copy can be obtained with purchase of source book)
Strengths Self-Assessment Questionnaire	Cognitive and appraisal skills Defences and coping mechanisms Temperamental and dispositional factors Interpersonal skills and supports External factors	38 scaled items	No cost

Recovery

The current emphasis on 'recovery' has emerged from the lived experience of people with mental illness which suggests that many individuals are able to overcome their difficulties to lead satisfying and contributing lives (Deegan, 1996). This clearly challenges the belief that conditions such as schizophrenia follow a course of progressive deterioration. Common themes in patient accounts of their recovery indicate that recovery involves developing new meaning and purpose in life, taking responsibility for one's illness, renewing a sense of hope, being involved in meaningful activities, managing symptoms, overcoming stigma and being supported by others (Davidson *et al.*, 2005; Deegan, 1996). Recovery in the mental health context does not necessarily mean 'cure' but implies that while individuals with mental illness may continue to experience symptoms and functional impairment, they can move beyond the negative consequences of the illness to achieve greater self-confidence and hope for the future. The concept of recovery provides a fresh approach to the provision of mental health services and is now widely promoted in most developed countries (Anthony, 1993).

While there is currently a growing number of measures designed to assess different aspects of recovery, these tend to be divided into (i) instruments that assess recovery from the perspective of the individual with mental illness, and (ii) instruments that assess the recovery orientation of the mental health services/provider. The measures of recovery included in this chapter focus on recovery from the perspective of the individual. The selection of these recovery measures was guided by the recent review of such measures conducted by Burgess and colleagues (2011). The group used strict selection criteria to short-list measures suitable for routine use with mental health clients. Two of the candidate measures shortlisted by the group, the Recovery Assessment Scale and the Illness Management and Recovery Scales, are described below. Based on the criteria employed by Burgess and colleagues (2011), these two measures assess domains related to personal recovery, are brief, take a client perspective, are suitable for use in routine practice, demonstrate sound psychometric properties and are acceptable to clients.

Recovery Assessment Scale

The Recovery Assessment Scale (RAS) was developed in the US by Giffort and colleagues (1995) and is now the most widely used self-report recovery scale for individuals with mental illness (Chiba *et al.*, 2010). The RAS was designed to assess the recovery process of individuals with serious and persistent mental illness. Two versions of the measure are currently available: the original 41-item version (Giffort *et al.*, 1995) and a brief 24-item version (Chiba *et al.*, 2010; Corrigan *et al.*, 2004).

Both versions assess (the same) five domains of recovery that are grounded in the experiences of those with mental illness. All statements are rated on a five-point scale (1 = strongly disagree to 5 = strongly agree) to provide a quantitative assessment of recovery. A total scale score is derived from summing the item scores for all items (Table 4.2). Higher scores represent higher self-reported levels of recovery.

Both versions of the measure are easy to score and have sound psychometric properties (Chiba *et al.*, 2010; Corrigan *et al.*, 2004; McNaught *et al.*, 2007). Prior research found a test-retest reliability of $r = 0.88$ between two administrations 14 days apart and convergent validity with the Empowerment Scale (Rogers *et al.*, 1997). The measure is self-completed by the client and no specific training of the client or person administering

Table 4.2   Example of Recovery Assessment Scale items and structure.

	Strongly disagree (1)	Disagree (2)	Not sure (3)	Agree (4)	Strongly agree (5)
I have goals in life that I want to reach	☐	☐	☐	☐	☐
I am the person most responsible for my own improvement	☐	☐	☐	☐	☐

the scale is required. The 24-item version of the measure takes 5–10 minutes to complete and yields valuable information for programme evaluation and treatment planning. Information concerning the factor structure of the 41-item version of the measure can be found at: http://schizophreniabulletin.oxfordjournals.org/content/30/4/1005/.full.pdf. Copies of the 24-item version (and information concerning reliability and validity of the measure) can be obtained from the publication by Chiba and colleagues (2010).

Illness Management and Recovery Scales

The Illness Management and Recovery (IMR) scales (Mueser *et al.*, 2004) were developed as a repeatable measure that quantifies a patient's progress towards management of their illness and achieving treatment goals. The IMR scales consider a number of illness management and recovery domains (personal goals, social supports, substance use, functioning, medication adherence, coping skills and participation in meaningful activities) rather than a single construct. The IMR scales have two versions, enabling the assessment of recovery from both practitioner and client perspectives (Table 4.3). Each version contains 15 items/statements, which are rated on a five-point Likert scale (ranging from 1 to 5). Higher scores represent higher self-reported levels of recovery.

A potential criticism of this measure is that a third of the items relate to more traditional clinical constructs associated with impairment, specifically medication adherence, symptom severity, impairment in functioning, relapse and psychiatric hospitalisation.

Empowerment

Despite the widespread use of the term in the mental health context, empowerment remains poorly understood (Corrigan, 2006). It has been defined as the level of personal control an individual has over important areas of their life, including not only mental health but also vocation, accommodation and relationships (Segal *et al.*, 1995). Empowerment is also closely related to autonomy which is also supported as a recovery ideal.

Empowerment is widely discussed and promoted by client groups and practitioners working in the rehabilitation field. Indeed, it is a key goal of most rehabilitation programmes for those with serious mental illness. Empowerment can be viewed from a

Table 4.3 Illness Management and Recovery (IMR) Scales.

	1	2	3	4	5
Client version – Progress towards personal goals					
In the past 3 months, I have come up with….	No personal goals	A personal goal, but have not done anything to finish my goal	A personal goal and made a little way towards finishing it	A personal goal and have gotten pretty far in finishing my goal	A personal goal and have finished it
Informant/practitioner version – Progress towards personal goals					
Please circle the option that fits your client the best. In the past 3 months, s/he has come up with ….	No personal goals	A personal goal, but has not done anything to finish their goal	A personal goal and made a little way towards finishing it	A personal goal and has gotten pretty far in finishing their goal	A personal goal and has finished it

broader treatment, organisational or community perspective. This might include activities such as involvement in decision making regarding one's own treatment or on committees of public mental health services or participation in mental health advocacy groups in the community. These perspectives are also highly consistent with recovery perspectives and have specific measures (e.g. treatment empowerment; see Hudon *et al.*, 2010), but here we limit ourselves to assessment of perceived empowerment around control of one's life at an individual level.

It is clear that empowerment is closely related to strengths and recovery-based practice in that a focus on recovery and strengths is likely to enhance empowerment. However, there is a paucity of measures devoted to the assessment of empowerment in the mental health field. One exception is the Making Decisions Empowerment Scale developed in the US by Young and Ensing (1999). The measure is described in greater detail below.

Making Decisions Empowerment Scale

The Making Decisions Empowerment Scale (commonly called the Empowerment Scale) was developed by a group of mental health clients with input from academics and researchers (Rogers *et al.*, 1997). The measure employs 28 statements/items that can be collapsed into five domains related to client empowerment. Items are rated on a four-point Likert scale (ranging from 1 = strongly agree to 4 = strongly disagree) with no 'neutral' option (Table 4.4). Item scores are summed and averaged to provide domain scores and an overall scale score. Higher scores indicate greater levels of perceived empowerment. Reliability coefficients for the scale range from 0.73 to 0.85 (Strack *et al.*, 2007).

Since 2003, the Ohio Department of Mental Health has included the Making Decisions Empowerment Scale in the suite of measures used to assess client outcomes. Copies of the scale can be obtained from the Department's website at: www.mh.state.oh.us/assets/client-outcomes/instruments/english-adult-client.pdf (refer to Section 4 for the items that make up the Empowerment Scale).

Table 4.4 Empowerment Scale: example of items/structure and scoring.

Please read each statement carefully and indicate the degree to which you agree or disagree with each item by placing a check mark in the appropriate box	Strongly disagree (1)	Disagree (2)	Agree (3)	Strongly agree (4)
I generally accomplish what I set out to do	☐	☐	☐	☐
I can pretty much determine what will happen in my life	☐	☐	☐	☐

Information concerning scoring and norms can be obtained from the website at: http://www.mh.state.oh.us/oper/outcomes/outcomes.index.html.

Strengths

Traditional assessment of individuals with mental illness tend to concentrate on identifying symptoms, problem behaviours and impairments. This problem-focused approach can have a negative impact on clients who frequently have difficulties with self-esteem and confidence following years of struggling with the symptoms of their illness. Further, problem-focused approaches often fail to consider more positive aspects such as client talents and abilities (Glover, 2005; Tedeschi & Kilmer, 2005). The 'strengths' approach suggests that individuals can learn from their problems as well as their successes. Thus, the approach tries to balance deficits in functioning with the abilities and strengths of the individual (Rapp & Goscha, 2006).

The definition of strengths is fairly broad and is relative to the capabilities of the individual rather than some comparison to others. Therefore, we introduce the concept of strengths to clients as 'assets' they have acquired which are all those things that help them deal with challenges and live the life they want to lead. We also include attitudes and values they hold as well as skills and abilities. Working with clients to identify their strengths may help practitioners obtain a better understanding of the resources that clients can draw on during their recovery.

In effect, the strengths approach aims to assist clients to use their skills, knowledge, talents and experience to achieve their goals. While the assessment of these constructs may appear to be a straightforward process, in reality it can be a difficult task (Cowger, 1994). Many clients do not recognise their strengths because historically there has been a focus on their problems or deficits or because they mistakenly believe that a strength requires that they excel in some domain. As a result, some discussion about the meaning of strengths is often helpful as part of the assessment process in order to broaden clients' perspective on what can be considered. Then a systematic approach, based on collaboration with the client, is required to tease out those qualities associated with coping and resilience (McQuaide & Ehrenreich, 1997).

The assessment of strengths has been undertaken through (i) informal, qualitative methods of assessment and (ii) the use of more structured quantitative approaches. The most widely used qualitative approach is the Strengths Assessment Worksheet developed by Rapp and Goscha (2006). Quantitative approaches involving scales and questionnaires are also popular. In this review we also discuss the Strengths Assessment Questionnaire (McQuaide & Ehrenreich, 1997).

Strengths Assessment Worksheet

The Worksheet is designed to help the practitioner and client to organise and record the multiple strengths that individuals possess. The Worksheet is completed via semi-structured interview with the client. Information is collected in a conversational manner around seven domains (daily living situation, financial/insurance, vocation/education,

Table 4.5   Example of Strengths Assessment Worksheet.

Current status – (*What are my current strengths?*)	Individual's desires/aspirations (*What do I want?*)	Resources, personal and social (*What strengths have I used in the past?*)
Daily living situation		
Document strengths here	*Document desires here*	*Document strengths used in the past here*

social support, health, leisure/recreation, spirituality/culture). The information is recorded in three key areas: current status, desires/aspirations and resources (Table 4.5).

The middle column of the Worksheet asks the question 'What do I want?'. This is at the heart of rehabilitation work and articulating this client dream or aspiration is critical to moving recovery forward. This part of the Worksheet can often connect with underlying values which are also a rich source of potential strengths. For example, if someone indicates that they would like more friends and they value relationships with others, this can prompt exploration of what it is about 'relationships' that is important to them and what they bring to a relationship. This might include potential strengths such as humour, reliability, being a good listener, loyalty, kindness, patience, etc. From the middle column, a list of priorities can be distilled and work can begin on a chosen goal.

It may take considerable time and a number of meetings to gain useful information for the completion of the Worksheet. The aim is to gain information that is genuine and meaningful to the client rather than simply what they think that you want to hear. Over time, strengths will become apparent, be noted and begin to populate the Worksheet. At first, the tool may lack detail but with increasing engagement with the client, it will become more specific and complete.

In practice, we have found that some clients have difficulty spontaneously coming up with strengths. There are several strategies that we have found useful in helping them become more aware of their strengths. Firstly, we ask them to think about how they spend their days and what they do when they have a 'good' day. Often having them reflect on a specific day of the week helps. Asking them what they did and what contributed to the experience of that day being 'positive' helps reveal strengths. If they are still having difficulties, we have found that providing a list of strengths helps since recognition is often easier than generation of strengths for some. Alternatively, there are specific questions that can help reveal strengths, e.g. how would you like someone to describe you? What are you most proud of?

Unlike most scaled measures that produce a numerical score, the Strengths Assessment Worksheet produces textural data. This is not especially useful in assessing change in clients over time. However, some of the other measures described in this chapter (e.g. the Recovery Assessment Scale and/or the Empowerment Scale) could be used in conjunction with the Strengths Assessment Worksheet to monitor change.

A copy of the Strengths Assessment Worksheet and information concerning its development are available from the publication by Rapp and Goscha (2006).

Table 4.6   Strengths Self-Assessment Questionnaire: examples of items and structure.

	Strongly disagree (1)	Disagree (2)	Not sure (3)	Agree (4)	Strongly agree (5)
4. I can anticipate a problem and come up with a plan to solve it	☐	☐	☐	☐	☐
14. My sense of humour helps me deal with stressful situations	☐	☐	☐	☐	☐

Strengths Self-Assessment Questionnaire

The Strengths Self-Assessment Questionnaire was developed in the USA by McQuaide and Ehrenreich (1997). The authors conducted a review of the literature to identify client characteristics associated with 'strengths' in individuals with mental illness. A large pool of characteristics was isolated and these were subsequently collapsed into five categories: cognitive and appraisal skills; defences and coping mechanisms; temperamental and dispositional factors; interpersonal skills and supports; and external factors. A self-report measure was then developed using key statements that seemed to represent each of these categories (Table 4.6).

While the questionnaire contains 38 statements, some aspects (such as cognitive abilities and locus of control) are not included as the developers of the scale felt that these would be better assessed through other means. The developers were also concerned that inclusion of sufficient items to assess these domains would make the scale too long and cumbersome. The 38 items are rated by the client using a five-point scale ('strongly disagree' to 'strongly agree'). It should be noted that the Strengths Self-Assessment Questionnaire is a clinical instrument, not a psychometrically validated instrument. As noted by McQuaide and Ehrenreich (1997), it is intended to '*alert the client and the worker to areas of perceived strength*' (p.208). A copy of the Strengths Self-Assessment Questionnaire and information concerning its development are available from the publication by McQuaide and Ehrenreich (1997).

Sam: assessing recovery, empowerment and strengths

Sam has been compliant with medications and his symptoms (i.e. hallucinations and delusions) have settled. However, he seems to be continually focused on how the illness destroyed his life and he believes that he will never be able to achieve anything worthwhile. You decide to conduct a strengths assessment using the Strengths Assessment Worksheet (Rapp, 1998). You feel that the act of completing the assessment will help Sam to recognise positive aspects of his life that may not have been apparent to him. Over the next couple of visits to Sam, you use semi-structured interviews to complete the Strengths Assessment Worksheet. During these interviews, Sam described his previous interest in music and how he played guitar at school. He now wants to start playing again and with your help, he has identified some goals such as checking out the cost of guitars, where to get lessons, local music groups, etc. Strengths identified include his interest in music, his ability to focus and concentrate when practising and his 'good ear for music'. An added strength and resource relates to Sam's recollection that he often felt more relaxed, calmer and 'less stressed' when he was practising guitar. Goals related to playing guitar again have been summarised under the 'leisure' domain on the Worksheet. A number of other goals have been identified in other domains and Sam's progress towards achieving these will be monitored on a regular basis.

Although Sam feels positive that he can achieve the goals identified, you are concerned that his low self-esteem may affect his ability to achieve these goals. You discuss this with Sam and he agrees to complete the Empowerment Scale (Rogers *et al*., 1997). The completed measure provides insights into five domains of empowerment. A summary of the data indicates that Sam has a significantly lower score on the 'optimism and control over future' subscale. Domains receiving low mean scores could be noted in Sam's care plan and become the focus of attention for you and Sam. These low-scoring domains may require additional input to improve Sam's perception of his ability to influence change in these areas.

Sam has been progressing well with the task of achieving his goals (identified during the strengths assessment). A recent assessment using the Empowerment Scale indicates that his sense of control over his life has been improving as indicated by the higher total scale score. Over the next week, you ask Sam to complete the brief 24-item version of the Recovery Assessment Scale (Chiba *et al*., 2010; Corrigan *et al*., 2004). You find that Sam has a significantly lower score on the 'Personal Confidence' subscale compared to the other four subscales. This is in keeping with the data obtained from the earlier assessment using the Empowerment Scale. Building confidence and self-efficacy in Sam will now become key elements of his rehabilitation plan.

Sam was able to purchase a second-hand guitar. Although he was frustrated by how slowly he progressed, he continued to enjoy practising. He also began more purposefully playing when he was 'feeling stressed' and he said this helped him feel 'more chilled'.

Summary

It is becoming increasingly clear that those employed in the rehabilitation field need to consider the use of a range of assessment measures with clients such as Sam. From the limited pool of measures available, we have identified a subset of strategies and measures that could be used to assess recovery, empowerment and strengths. It should be noted that these are at different stages of development. Aspects such as normative data are not yet available. However, normative data are not essential for these measures since they are individualised measures (ideographic) that can be used to reveal the unique capabilities or potential of clients that can be assessed over time.

Use of the measures described will provide valuable insights into how individuals such as Sam view their goals and their ability to achieve these in the future. This information can be used in goal setting and the planning of rehabilitation programmes. Engaging the client in the process of assessing these domains sends a clear message that empowerment and strengths are important aspects of the journey towards recovery. Instead of focusing on the 'things' that individuals cannot do, the process of assessing domains such as strengths will help clients to identify positive aspects of their persona. This exercise is likely to combat the negative aspects of the illness and give clients a sense of hope for the future.

References

Anthony W (1993) Recovery from mental illness: the guiding vision of the mental health service system in the 1990s. *Psychosocial Rehabilitation Journal* **12**, 55–81.

Burgess P, Pirkis J, Coombs T, Rosen A (2011) Assessing the value of existing recovery measures for routine use in Australian mental health services. *Australian and New Zealand Journal of Psychiatry* **45**, 267–80.

Chiba R, Miyamoto Y, Kawakami N (2010) Reliability and validity of the Japanese version of the Recovery Assessment Scale (RAS) for people with chronic mental illness: scale development. *International Journal of Nursing Studies* **47**, 314–22.

Corrigan P (2006) Impact of client operated services on empowerment and recovery of people with psychiatric disabilities. *Psychiatric Services* **57**, 1493–6.

Corrigan P, Salzer M, Ralph R, Sangster Y, Keck L (2004) Examining the factor structure of the Recovery Assessment Scale. *Schizophrenia Bulletin* **30**, 1035–41.

Cowger C (1994) Assessing client strengths: clinical assessment for empowerment. *Social Work* **39**, 262–8.

Davidson L, Sells D, Sangster S, O'Connell M (2005) Qualitative studies of recovery: what can we learn from the person? In: Corrigan P, Ralph R (eds) *Recovery in Mental Illness: Broadening Our Understanding*. American Psychological Society: Washington, DC, pp.147–70.

Deegan P (1996) Recovery as a journey of the heart. *Psychiatric Rehabilitation Journal* **19**, 91–7.

Giffort D, Schmook A, Woody C, Vollendorf C, Gervain M (1995) *Recovery Assessment Scale*. Illinois Department of Mental Health: Chicago, IL.

Glover H (2005) Recovery based service delivery: are we ready to transform the words into a paradigm shift? *Australian e-Journal for the Advancement of Mental Health* **4**, 1–4.

Hasson-Ohayon I, Roe D, Kravetz S (2007) A randomised controlled trial of the effectiveness of the Illness Management and Recovery Program. *Psychiatric Services* **58**, 1461–6.

Hudon C, St-Cyr Tribble D, Legare F, Bravo G, Fortin M, Almirall J (2010) Assessing enablement in clinical practice: a systematic review of available instruments. *Journal of Evaluation in Clinical Practice* **16**, 1301–8.

McNaught M, Caputi P, Oades L, Deane F (2007) Testing the validity of the Recovery Assessment Scale using an Australian sample. *Australian and New Zealand Journal of Psychiatry* **41**, 450–7.

McQuaide S, Ehrenreich J (1997) Assessing client strengths. *Families in Society* **78**, 201–12.

Mueser K, Gingerich S, Salyers M, McGuire A, Reyes R, Cunningham H (2004) *The Illness Management and Recovery (IMR) Scales (Client and Practitioner Versions)*. Dartmouth Psychiatric Research Center: Concord, NH.

Rapp C (1998) *The Strengths Model: Case Management with People Suffering from Severe and Persistent Mental Illness*. Oxford University Press: London.

Rapp C, Goscha R (2006) *The Strengths Model: Case Management with People with Psychiatric Disabilities*, 2nd edn. Oxford University Press: Oxford.

Rogers ES, Chamberlin J, Ellison ML, Crean T (1997) A client-constructed scale to measure empowerment among users of mental health services. *Psychiatric Services* **48**, 1042–7.

Segal S, Silverman C, Temkin T (1995) Measuring empowerment in client-run self-help agencies. *Community Mental Health Journal* **31**, 215–27.

Strack K, Deal W, Schlenberg S (2007) Coercion and empowerment in the treatment of individuals with serious mental illness. A preliminary investigation. *Psychological Services* **4**, 96–106.

Tedeschi R, Kilmer R (2005) Assessing strengths, resilience and growth to guide clinical interventions. *Professional Psychology* **36**, 230–7.

Young SL, Ensing DS (1999) Exploring recovery from the perspective of people with psychiatric disabilities. *Psychiatric Rehabilitation Journal* **22**, 219–31.

Chapter 5

Assessing Quality of Life and Perceptions of Care

Tom Meehan and William Brennan

> You have engaged Sam and a group of other people with severe mental illness in a rehabilitation programme. You hope that they are finding the programme worthwhile and that it is making a positive contribution to their quality of life. You are looking for measures that will give you reliable feedback on how the clients are experiencing the programme and some means of monitoring changes in their quality of life.

While symptoms and impairment may continue to affect the lives of individuals such as Sam, perceptions of one's quality of life may alter over time. Indeed, improvement in quality of life is frequently considered the ultimate goal of rehabilitation services for individuals with severe and persistent mental illness (Oliver *et al.*, 1996). However, traditional measures of outcome for those with severe mental illness have generally relied on the assessment of symptoms and impairment. While these indicators are important, they tend to be limited and fail to consider broader quality of life issues such as accommodation, finances, employment, physical health, leisure, social relations, etc. It is now clear that any assessment of people with psychiatric disability needs to consider quality of life and satisfaction (in addition to symptoms and functioning).

There is lack of agreement, however, on what factors should be considered when assessing quality of life in the mental health field. Nonetheless, it is generally accepted that quality of life is multidimensional and measures should include some assessment of the domains described above. Moreover, it is also clear that assessment of quality of life should include an *objective* component (such as the amount of money one has to spend) and a *subjective* component (i.e. how the individual feels about the amount of money they have to spend). In this chapter, we focus on quality of life measures that meet the criteria discussed above. Moreover, the selected measures have been found to be useful in clients with severe mental illness (e.g. Wisconsin Quality of Life Index and the Quality of Life Self-Assessment Inventory) and in those displaying deficit syndrome (e.g. Quality of Life Scale) (Table 5.1).

Manual of Psychosocial Rehabilitation, First Edition. Edited by Robert King, Chris Lloyd, Tom Meehan, Frank P. Deane and David J. Kavanagh.
© 2012 Blackwell Publishing Ltd. Published 2012 by Blackwell Publishing Ltd.

Table 5.1 Summary of measures.

Measure	Domains assessed	Administration	Cost
Assessment of quality of life			
WHOQOL-BREF (WHOQOL Group, 1998)	Physical Psychological Social relationships Environment	Self-report or semi-structured interview with client (26 items)	No cost
Quality of Life Self-Assessment Inventory (Skantze et al., 1992)	Housing Housing environment Household and self-care Knowledge and education Leisure Physical health Contacts Work Inner experience Community service Dependence	Self-report by client (100 items)	No cost
Wisconsin Quality of Life Index (W-QLI) (Becker et al., 1993)	Life satisfaction Occupational activities Psychological wellbeing Physical health Social relations Finances Activities of daily living Symptoms Patient's own goals	Three versions: - consumer (42 items) - carers/family (28 items) - practitioner (68 items)	No cost
Quality of Life Scale(QLS) (Heinrichs et al., 1984)	Intrapsychic foundations Interpersonal relations Instrumental role category Common objectives and activities	Semi-structured interview with client (21 items)	No cost
Assessment of satisfaction			
Satisfaction with Daily Occupations (SDO) (Eklund, 2004)	Work Leisure Domestic tasks Self-care	Interview with client (9 items)	No cost
Inpatient Evaluation of Satisfaction Questionnaire (IESQ) (Meehan et al., 2002)	Staff–patient alliance Treatment Hospital environment	Self-report or with assistance from carer/practitioner (22 items)	No cost
Verona Service Satisfaction Scale – European Version (Ruggeri et al., 2000)	Overall satisfaction Professionals' skills and behaviour Information Access Efficacy Types of intervention Relative's involvement	Self-report or with assistance from practitioner (54 items)	Permission Required

   Client satisfaction with the services received is also becoming increasingly important. Satisfaction has been found to be important in influencing other client outcomes in that more satisfied clients demonstrate better outcomes (Ruggeri, 1994). Methods of assessing satisfaction have steadily improved over the past 20 years and there is now a range of measures available for assessing satisfaction in different health care settings, including mental health. The measures discussed in this chapter can be administered by interview (Satisfaction with Daily Occupations) or through self-report (Inpatient Evaluation of Satisfaction Questionnaire and Verona Service Satisfaction Scale). Moreover, they are brief, easy to score and have adequate psychometric properties (see Table 5.1).

   While other quality of life and satisfaction measures are available, these tend to be too long and cumbersome for use in individuals with severe mental illness.

Quality of life

As outlined earlier, improving one's quality of life is an important component of rehabilitation efforts. For many individuals with severe disability, return to full functioning may not be possible. However, being able to live a full and satisfying life within the limitations of one's disabilities may be a realistic goal for many. Below, we discuss four quality of life measures that could be considered for use in clients with severe and persistent mental illness.

World Health Organization Quality of Life (Brief Version)

The original version of the World Health Organization Quality of Life (WHOQOL) measure was developed by a multinational group seeking a measure that would capture cultural issues in addition to the usual quality of life domains (WHOQOL Group, 1998). The original version of the measure contains 100 statements/items and assesses six quality of life domains (physical health, psychological health, level of independence, social relationships, environment and spirituality). More recently, a brief version of the measure (WHOQOL-BREF) containing 26 items has emerged (Skevington et al., 2004). The 26-item version provides assessment of four domains (physical, psychological, social and environmental). Items are rated on the degree to which one experiences a number of given activities and satisfaction with aspects of life (Box 5.1).

   The WHOQOL-BREF can be completed through self-report (5 minutes) or practitioner interview (15–20 minutes). While the instrument is easy to understand and complete, the

Box 5.1 WHOQOL-BREF: example of items					
How much do you enjoy life?	Not at all	A little	A moderate amount	Very much	An extreme amount
How satisfied are you with your health?	Very dissatisfied	Dissatisfied	Neither satisfied nor dissatisfied	Satisfied	Very satisfied

scoring is somewhat complicated in that three items (Q3, Q4, Q26) are reverse scored prior to calculation of domain scores and total score. Raw scores are then transformed to a scale of 0–100. The manual that accompanies the measure will assist practitioners in this task.

The University of Bath is the WHO distributor for the UK version. Users must register to use the measure and this can be done online at: www.bath.ac.uk/whoqol/questionnaire/info.cfm. Copies of all WHOQOL measures are also available from the site at no cost.

Wisconsin Quality of Life Index

The Wisconsin Quality of Life Index (W-QLI) was developed in the US by Becker and colleagues (1993). The measure differs from others in the mental health field in that it was developed for use in those with severe and persistent mental illness (Becker *et al.*, 1993). The measure is one of the most comprehensive available since it covers nine quality of life domains and provides ratings from three key players: the client, his/her carer and his/her service provider. The W-QLI scores range from -3 (the worst things could be) to +3 (the best things could be). A score of 0 on the W-QLI is a middle-range score which is close to the average or normative value for the target population. Each domain is scored separately using a combination of satisfaction and importance scores (Box 5.2). When W-QLI scores are computer scored, a one-page report is produced documenting the score for each domain. Client goals for improvement with treatment are presented verbatim, allowing the clients and service providers to discuss discrepancies and come to agreement on goals to be pursued.

The W-QLI is an easy-to-use self-report or practitioner-administered instrument used to assess and monitor quality of life in individuals with severe mental illness. It is designed to document client goals for improvement with treatment and to aid clients and staff in their work together to achieve desired goals and improved quality of life for clients. The developers of the measure (Becker *et al.*, 1993) report that through use of the measure:

- clients and providers will increase their understanding of the current client quality of life status
- clients will take a more active role in their treatment
- communication between clients and providers will be improved
- the practitioner's role as client educator will be enhanced
- clients will increase their quality of life and goal achievement, leading to increased empowerment.

Box 5.2   Wisconsin Quality of Life Index: example of items

How do you feel about your physical health? (Check one)
☐ Very dissatisfied ☐ Moderately dissatisfied ☐ A little dissatisfied
☐ Neither satisfied or dissatisfied
☐ A little satisfied ☐ Moderately satisfied ☐ Very satisfied

How important to you is your physical health? (Check one)
☐ Not at all important ☐ Slightly important ☐ Moderately important
☐ Very important ☐ Extremely important

The measure also has the advantage of capturing multiple views of a client's quality of life (client, provider and carer). Differences between the ratings indicate the need for discussion with the different parties to identify the reason for such differences. This provides an opportunity to enhance the working alliance between clients and providers/ carers. The psychometric properties of the measure are adequate (Diaz *et al.*, 1999; Sainfort *et al.*, 1996).

Notwithstanding the above advantages, the measure is relatively long (takes about 25 minutes to complete the client version) and it has a variety of response options (as outlined in the sample item in Box 5.2. As such, it would prove difficult to apply the measure via telephone interview. Moreover, it is more difficult to score than the other measures reviewed. However, a computer program is available to assist with scoring.

General information about the W-QLI is provided at the W-QLI website at http://wqli. fmhi.usf.edu. Copies of the measure and the scoring manual are available free of cost. However, the user needs to sign a copyright agreement and provide deidentified data to Professor Becker for ongoing testing of the measure. Email address for Professor Becker is: becker@fmhi.usf.edu.

Quality of Life Self-Assessment Inventory

The Quality of Life Self-Assessment Inventory (QLS-100) was developed in the UK by Skantze and colleagues (1992). It contains 100 factors which are organised under 11 quality of life domains. For example, the 'Housing' domain contains the following factors: size, lighting, heating, hot water, drinking water, kitchen, toilet, bath/shower, appearance, peace and privacy. To complete the measure, individuals simply circle those aspects/ factors which are considered unsatisfactory in their life (Box 5.3). The number of factors circled is subtracted from the total number (i.e. 100) to provide a scale score. A lower score indicates that more items have been circled and this implies that the individual has more factors requiring attention and, as such, a lower quality of life. A 7-day test-retest reliability for the measure total score was high with a correlation coefficient of $r = 0.88$.

This measure is one of the easiest to complete and one of the least difficult to score. Items identified by clients as being unsatisfactory can become the focus of further discussion with the individuals involved. In the example provided in Box 5.3, 'clothing' has been circled/identified as being unsatisfactory by the client. Further questioning of the client is required to identify what aspects of his/her clothing are considered unsatisfactory and what interventions are required to address this.

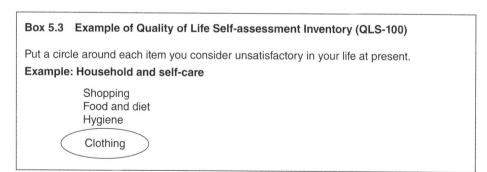

Box 5.3   Example of Quality of Life Self-assessment Inventory (QLS-100)

Put a circle around each item you consider unsatisfactory in your life at present.
Example: Household and self-care

       Shopping
       Food and diet
       Hygiene

       Clothing

While this method of assessing quality of life is likely to maximise the relevance of quality of life measurement for the individual, it can be difficult to compare results between individuals (and services) since the ratings refer to personally defined items/domains which are likely to vary between individuals. For example, two clients receiving a total scale score of 80 may have selected different items from the scale and thus hold very different views of the factors affecting their quality of life.

The measure is available in the publication by Skantze and Malm (1994).

Quality of Life Scale

The Quality of Life Scale (QLS) was developed in the USA to provide a measure of functioning/quality of life in individuals with schizophrenia (Heinrichs *et al.*, 1984). It is particularly useful in this client group as it has a strong focus on assessment of deficit/negative symptoms. The QLS contains 21 items (19 rated on a seven-point scale and two rated on a five-point scale) using information collected via semi-structured interview (Box 5.4). The interviewer is encouraged to ask questions around each item until adequate information is available to make a judgement about the score to be selected. Each domain comes with a set of possible probe questions to elicit the information required to score that domain (see Box 5.4). While information is provided to assist with selecting a score, this information is only available for every other option. Subscales/domain scores can be obtained by summing item scores for a given domain and dividing by the number of items in that domain. Higher scores represent higher functioning/quality of life.

Although the measure has only 21 items, it takes about 45 minutes to administer due to the need to collect sufficient information from the client to rate the measure. Moreover, the measure is designed to be rated by mental health practitioners or staff with training. It is not suitable for inpatients but could be used at the time of admission to assess negative symptoms and functioning in those being admitted. It has good inter-rater

---

Box 5.4   Quality of Life Scale: example of item

This item is to rate the extent to which the person is unable to initiate or sustain goal-directed activity due to inadequate drive.

Suggested questions:
How have you been going about accomplishing your goals? What other things have you worked on or accomplished lately? Have there been tasks in any area that you wanted to do but didn't because you somehow didn't get around to it? How motivated have you been? Do you have much enthusiasm, energy, and drive? Have you tended to get into a rut? Have you tended to put things off?

0- Lack of motivation
1-
2- Able to meet basic maintenance demands of life but lack of motivation significantly impairs any progress or new accomplishments
3-
4- Able to meet routine demands of life and some new accomplishments, but lack of motivation results in significant underachievement in some areas
5-
6- No evidence of significant lack of motivation

reliability and good convergent validity with the Lehman Quality of Life Interview (Lehman *et al.*, 1993). The measure can be used at no cost but permission to use it needs to be obtained from:

Professor William T Carpenter
Maryland Psychiatric Research Center
PO Box 21247
Baltimore MD 21228, USA
email: wcarpent@mprc.umaryland.edu

Satisfaction

Client perceptions of the services received are now widely canvassed to provide information for the planning, delivery and evaluation of mental health services (Rey *et al.*, 1999). The increasing use of satisfaction surveys in the mental health field has been driven by the move towards client participation, the need to provide data for quality assurance/accreditation purposes and as a measure of treatment outcome (Parker *et al.*, 1996). Although there is no universally accepted method of assessing patient satisfaction, the use of self-completed questionnaires by patients is commonly employed.

Satisfaction with Daily Occupations

The Satisfaction with Daily Occupations (SDO) questionnaire was developed in Sweden and consists of nine items concerning satisfaction in four occupational areas (Eklund, 2004). These include work (four items concerning participation in work/rehab/community activities), leisure activities (two items concerning organised activities and independent activities), domestic tasks (two items concerning household chores, repairs/gardening) and self-care (one item). The questionnaire is administered via a semi-structured interview with the client. Each item consists of a two-part question. The first part queries whether or not the client presently performs the targeted activity. The second asks the client to rate his/her satisfaction with that activity on a seven-point scale from 1 = worst possible to 7 = best possible (Box 5.5).

Two scores are derived from the scale: one reflects the level of client engagement in daily activities (based on the 'yes'/'no' responses) and the second is a client satisfaction

---

Box 5.5   Satisfaction with Daily Occupations Scale: example of item

Work:

Item 2. [The client] has been in training/rehabilitation or has been studying during the past two months
Yes/No Note satisfaction score _____ (1–7)

Self-care:

Item 9. [The client] performs daily self-care (e.g. hygiene, care of hair, dressing)
Yes/No Note satisfaction score _____ (1–7)

score (derived from the rating on the 1–7 scale for each item). An overall satisfaction score can be obtained by summing the nine scaled items (range 0–63).

While the SDO is brief, it provides an assessment of the most important aspects of occupational functioning (work, leisure, domestic tasks and self-care). The scale is useful in that it engages the client in rating his/her own performance and satisfaction. In addition, the scale goes beyond the simple assessment of activity level (i.e. client engagement in activities) to provide a client satisfaction score for each activity. As a consequence, the SDO is likely to be useful in the rehabilitation field as a client outcome measure. However, further work on the ability of the scale to detect change over time ('sensitivity to change') is required. The SDO was developed using outpatient samples and it is unclear if it could be used for assessment of inpatients. As some interpretation of the scores is required, the SDO is best administered by professionally trained rehabilitation/clinical workers. While there is no cost associated with the use of the SDO, permission to use it should be sought from Professor Eklund:

Professor Mona Eklund
Professor of Occupational Therapy
Department of Health Sciences
Lund University
PO Box 157, SE-221 00
Lund, Sweden
email: mona.eklund@med.lu.se

Inpatient Evaluation of Service Questionnaire

The Inpatient Evaluation of Service Questionnaire (IESQ) was developed in Australia to provide a brief measure of satisfaction among inpatients (Meehan *et al.*, 2002). The item pool for the measure was derived from focus group discussions and individual interviews with clients approaching discharge from inpatient care. The 22 items in the main body of the questionnaire are rated on a five-point scale using the 'E5' response format (poor, fair, good, very good and excellent) suggested by Ware and Hays (1988). These categories offer greater variability across responses, particularly at the positive end of the scale (since individuals are mostly positive in their ratings of satisfaction) (Table 5.2). These 22 items can be collapsed into three domains: staff–patient alliance, treatment and environment. Cronbach's alpha for the three factors ranged from 0.78 to 0.93.

In addition to the 22 items in the main scale, two further items rate behavioural intentions (*advise a friend with similar problems to come to the hospital*, and *intent to return to the hospital if they had similar problems in the future*). Finally, two open-ended questions enable patients to provide qualitative feedback on aspects of their hospital stay that they 'liked most' and 'liked least'.

The IESQ was developed to provide a brief, user-friendly instrument that overcomes some of the shortcomings of existing satisfaction measures. It covers a broad range of inpatient concerns, is simply worded, easy to score and designed to be completed independently by the patient. While it assesses a number of satisfaction constructs,

Table 5.2   Inpatient Evaluation of Service Questionnaire: example of item.

Please take a few moments to think about your time in hospital. How would you rate the following?	Poor	Fair	Good	Very good	Excellent	Not sure
1 The **information** you received about **practical hospital matters** (e.g. meal times, smoking policy, money....)	□	□	□	□	□	□
11 The **attention** that staff gave to your worries and concerns	□	□	□	□	□	□

administration time is kept below 5 minutes. The measure has demonstrated ability to detect change in clients moving between inpatient services (Cleary *et al.*, 2003). Copies of the measure and information on scoring can be obtained from Dr Tom Meehan via email: Thomas_Meehan@health.qld.gov.au.

Verona Service Satisfaction Scale (European Version)

The Verona Service Satisfaction Scale (European Version) (VSSS-EU) was derived from the original 84-item version of the measure developed by Ruggeri and Dall'Agnola (1993). The 54 items yield seven dimensions which cover a wide range of factors related to satisfaction with inpatient and community mental health services. Items 1–40 are rated on a five-point scale ranging from 1= terrible to 5 = excellent. Each of the items between 41 and 54 is made up of three questions which enquire about receipt of specific interventions, was the individual satisfied with the intervention, and if they did not receive the intervention, would they have liked to receive the intervention? This provides a measure of satisfaction with the interventions provided and the decision by the mental health service not to provide an intervention, if that was the case (Ruggeri *et al.*, 2000).

The VSSS-EU was designed for self-administration by the client, thus eliminating the need for staff training. For clients with cognitive impairment, severe psychopathology and low level of literacy, a staff member could assist the client by reading the items to them. It takes approximately 20 minutes to administer the questionnaire and the rating period is the past 12 months. The measure has been shown to have good psychometric properties and is a reliable instrument for assessing satisfaction in individuals with schizophrenia (Ruggeri *et al.*, 2000). While this version of the measure was developed for use in cross-national studies, the measure could be used at the local level. However, the Professional Skills and Behaviour domain covers client satisfaction with a number of different providers such as nurses, social workers, psychologists, psychiatrists. This domain may prove difficult to rate for those clients receiving community treatment from a single case manager.

A copy of the VSSS-EU is available in the article by Ruggeri and colleagues (2000). Permission to use the measure should be obtained from:

Professor Mirella Ruggeri
Dipartimento di Medicina e Sanità Pubblica
Sezione di Psichiatria e di Psicologia Clinica, Università di
Verona, Policlinico G.B. Rossi
Piazzale L.A. Scuro 10
37134 Verona, Italy
email: mirella.ruggeri@univ.it

Using the measures in practice

Sam has been out of hospital and living independently in the community in his own apartment for the past 3 months. While the positive symptoms of his illness have settled, you notice that he is having great difficulty with deficit symptoms such as lack of motivation, poor emotional response and anhedonia (loss of sense of pleasure). You are interested in how Sam perceives these aspects of his functioning and would also like to have baseline data for ongoing monitoring. A review of quality of life measures indicates that the Quality of Life Scale (Heinrichs et al., 1984) would be useful as it is designed to assess deficit symptoms. A time is arranged with Sam to complete the measure. You work through each of the 21 items using a semi-structured interview approach. Subscales/domain scores are obtained by summing item scores for a given domain and dividing by the number of items in that domain. In Sam's case, the lowest mean score (mean = 2.30 out of a possible mean of 5) was found in the Intrapsychic Foundations domain (sense of purpose, motivation, curiosity, anhedonia, aimless inactivity, empathy, emotional interaction). Given that lower scores represent lower functioning/quality of life, it is clear that Sam will require additional assistance in providing him with a sense of purpose and examining strategies to improve his motivation.

Closely related to quality of life is the issue of satisfaction with mental health services and treatment. You review the available measures and decide to use the Satisfaction with Daily Occupations (SDO) questionnaire (Eklund, 2004) as it is brief (nine items) and covers areas important to Sam such as participation in community activities, leisure activities, domestic tasks and self-care. You administer the SDO during a semi-structured interview with Sam. He receives a score of 35 out of a possible 63. Further examination of the scores indicates that Sam is most dissatisfied with his participation in community activities. Increasing community activities will be highlighted in Sam's care plan and become a major goal of his rehabilitation programme. You will repeat the QLS and the SDO in 3 months to monitor change in these domains.

Summary

Since the 1970s, a range of measures has been introduced to assess quality of life and satisfaction. These vary significantly in relation to length, the domains assessed, the approach taken (interview versus self-report), scoring (a single scale score versus separate scores for each domain), training required, cost and time required to administer the measure. These factors need to be considered when selecting a measure for use with individuals who have severe mental illness.

References

Becker M, Diamond R, Sainfort F (1993) A new patient-focused index for measuring quality of life in persons with severe and persistent mental illness. *Quality of Life Research* **2**, 239–51.

Cleary M, Horsfall J, Hunt G (2003) Consumer feedback on nursing care and discharge planning. *Journal of Advanced Nursing* **42**, 269–77.

Diaz P, Mercier C, Hachey R, Caron J, Boyer G (1999) An evaluation of psychometric properties of the client's questionnaire of the Wisconsin Quality of Life Index-Canadian version (CaW-QLI). *Quality of Life Research* **8**, 509–14.

Eklund M (2004) Satisfaction with Daily Occupations: a tool for client evaluation in mental health care. *Scandinavian Journal of Occupational Therapy* **11**, 136–42.

Heinrichs D, Hanlon T, Carpenter W (1984) The Quality of Life Scale: an instrument for rating the schizophrenic deficit syndrome. *Schizophrenia Bulletin* **10**, 388–98.

Lehman AF (1988) A quality of life interview for the chronically mentally ill. *Evaluation and Program Planning* **11**, 51–62.

Lehman AF, Postrado LT, Rachuba LT (1993) Convergent validity of quality of life assessments for persons with severe mental illnesses. *Quality of Life Research* **2**, 327–33.

Meehan T, Bergen H, Stedman T (2002) Monitoring consumer satisfaction with inpatient care: the Inpatient Evaluation of Service Questionnaire. *Australian and New Zealand Journal of Psychiatry* **36**, 807–11.

Oliver J, Huxley P, Bridges K, Mohamad H (1996) *Quality of Life and Mental Health Services*. Routledge: London, pp.15–47.

Parker G, Wright M, Robertson S, Gladstone G (1996) The development of a patient satisfaction measure for psychiatric outpatients. *Australian and New Zealand Journal of Psychiatry* **30**, 343–9.

Rey J, Plapp J, Simpson P (1999) Parental satisfaction and outcome: a 4-year study in a child and adolescent mental health service. *Australian and New Zealand Journal of Psychiatry* **33**, 22–8.

Rugggeri M (1994) Patients' and relatives' satisfaction with psychiatric services: the state of the art of its measurement. *Social Psychiatry and Psychiatric Epidemiology* **29**, 212–27.

Ruggeri M, Dall'Agnola R (1993) The development and use of the Verona Expectations for Care Scale (VECS) and the Verona Service Satisfaction Scale (VSSS) for measuring expectations and satisfaction with community-based psychiatric services in patients, relatives and professionals. *Psychological Medicine* **23**, 511–23.

Ruggeri M, Lasalvia A, Dall'Agnola R *et al*. for the EPSILON Study Group (2000) Development, internal consistency and reliability of the Verona Service Satisfaction Scale – European Version. *British Journal of Psychiatry* **177**(Suppl), 41–8.

Sainfort F, Becker M, Diamond R (1996) Judgements of quality of life of individuals with severe mental disorders: patient self-report versus provider perspectives. *American Journal of Psychiatry* **153**, 497–501.

Skantze K, Malm U (1994) A new approach to facilitation of working alliances based on patients' quality of life goals. *Nordic Journal of Psychiatry* **48**, 37–55.

Skantze K, Malm U, Dencker S, May P, Corrigan P (1992) Comparison of quality of life with standard of living in schizophrenia outpatients. *British Journal of Psychiatry* **161**, 797–801.

Skevington S, Lofty M, O'Connell K (2004) WHOQOL Group: the World Health Organization's WHOQOL-BREF quality of life assessment: psychometric properties and results of the international field trial. *Quality of Life Research* **13**, 299–310.

Ware J, Hays R (1988) Methods for measuring patient satisfaction with specific medical encounters. *Medical Care* **26**, 393–402.

WHOQOL Group (1998) The World Health Organization Quality of Life assessment (WHOQOL): development and general psychometric properties. *Social Science and Medicine* **46**, 1569–85.

Part II
Therapeutic Skills and Interventions

Chapter 6

Deciding on Life Changes: The Role of Motivational Interviewing

Robert King and David J. Kavanagh

> Sam is a smoker. He was a late starter. He smoked his first cigarette in the 'smokers area' near to the outpatient clinic he was attending. He was chatting with another client of the service who offered him a smoke. He is not sure why but he accepted. He still does not know quite how he got into it, but these days it is a regular thing. He prefers to buy 'tailor-made' cigarettes but they are expensive and he always has a pouch of tobacco and some papers as well as some nicotine stains. He knows smoking is bad for his health and his doctors regularly remind him of the fact. However, his long-term health is not a major issue at the moment. The only times he ever thinks about trying to quit is when he runs out of money.

Population studies indicate that people with a mental illness are twice as likely to smoke as people with no mental illness (Lasser *et al.*, 2000). People with a diagnosis of schizophrenia have especially high rates of smoking (de Leon & Diaz, 2005; Ziedonis *et al.*, 2008). The reason why people with mental illness smoke more than the general population is unclear but it appears that some combination of the nicotine and the act of smoking provides some stimulation and/or comfort that alleviates some of the symptoms of mental illness. It is also likely that the high rate of smoking among people with severe mental illness normalizes it. Smoking is one of several lifestyle factors that have been identified as contributing to higher rates of physical illness and shorter lifespan among people with severe mental illness (de Hert *et al.*, 2011).

> Sam's smoking is unhealthy, but he does not appear motivated to change. Change will require motivation because most people find it difficult to stop smoking and people with chronic mental illness may find it more difficult than most. Sam's rehabilitation worker knows that telling Sam that smoking is unhealthy or 'nagging' him will not motivate him. Instead, she decides to use motivational interviewing (Miller & Rollnick, 2002; Rollnick *et al.*, 2008) as a strategic approach to engaging him and possibly increasing his motivation to change.

Manual of Psychosocial Rehabilitation, First Edition. Edited by Robert King, Chris Lloyd, Tom Meehan, Frank P. Deane and David J. Kavanagh.
© 2012 Blackwell Publishing Ltd. Published 2012 by Blackwell Publishing Ltd.

Three independent meta-analyses (de Leon & Diaz, 2010; Heckman *et al.*, 2010; Hettema & Hendricks, 2010) have found motivational interviewing to be effective, and probably more effective than other psychological interventions designed to assist people to quit smoking. Motivational interviewing is also effective in helping people with a range of other important lifestyle changes in areas such as alcohol use, substance use, weight loss and exercise.

Of particular relevance to Sam, interventions that assist people without mental illness to quit smoking have been found to have equal impact for people with severe mental illness, and there is no evidence that trying to quit worsens psychiatric symptoms (Banham & Gilbody, 2010). In addition, motivational interviewing has demonstrated a positive impact on other substance use by people with severe mental illness (Baker *et al.*, 2009; Kavanagh *et al.*, 2004), although the evidence for more sustained and wide-ranging treatment is somewhat stronger than that for brief interventions (Kavanagh & Mueser, 2010).

What is motivational interviewing?

Motivational interviewing (MI) creates conditions for change. MI is a brief intervention designed to provide conditions that accentuate existing motivations to change, and assist people to make their own decisions about change. It is not a tool to get people to change.

Motivational interviewing acknowledges that ambivalence about change is normal. It helps people work through the ambivalence and encourages their discussion of change and of core values. It increases their confidence in making a change, by helping them remember other self-control challenges they were successful in meeting. When they do decide to make a positive lifestyle change, MI helps them turn intentions into sustained action, by creating a detailed plan.

Motivational interviewing is not a programmatic therapy. It is about engaging the person in rehabilitation or in changing their behaviour, and can therefore be used in brief interventions (e.g. 1–2 sessions) or woven into an extended rehabilitation programme. When used thematically in rehabilitation, its focus is on maintaining or regaining motivation and engagement, as well as on initial engagement. While its focus is on the person's own motivation, the approach has also been adapted for use in groups. In that case, individuals are encouraged to consider whether ideas presented by other group members also apply to them.

Empathy and warmth are at its core; confrontation is not used. MI was originally derived from Bill Miller's observation that therapist empathy was a strong predictor of change in problem drinkers (Miller & Baca, 1983), which in turn reflected an influence of Carl Rogers' therapeutic approach (Rogers, 1959). This led Miller to develop MI as an approach to development of motivation, culminating in the first book on the topic with Stephen Rollnick (1991) and its later edition in 2002.

Empathy and warmth help the person feel safe to acknowledge problems with their current behaviour: empathy for problems can also help to augment their emotional impact. On the other hand, confrontation undermines the therapeutic relationship and tends to elicit withdrawal from the situation or defensive arguments for the status quo. These arguments have the effect of increasing commitment to the dysfunctional behaviour. So, if a client resists change, an MI practitioner avoids putting pressure on them and gives them the option to stop the discussion (deflecting or 'rolling with' resistance).

Motivational interviewing encourages clients to talk about change. MI tries to reverse the usual roles, where a practitioner is trying to convince a person to change. Instead, MI encourages clients to talk about change: about the benefits it may bring and about its possibility.

Motivational interviewing is person centred. While MI has an agenda, it is the person's own motivations that are elicited. So, it encourages the client to do most of the talking. In practice, practitioners often find it hard to adapt their practice to this approach, and may confuse the approach with clinical assessments, which tend to use convergent questions (e.g. 'Have you been coughing a lot in the mornings lately?') to provide a comprehensive examination of symptoms. In MI, the person is encouraged to explore their experiences (e.g. '… any health issues that could be related to smoking?'). MI does not necessarily cover every potential problem: It is about the issues that are salient for that person.

Motivational interviewing is about emotional reactions. In essence, MI acknowledges that motivation is about emotional reactions: anticipated pleasure, worries or concerns about unwanted outcomes. Salient benefits or costs tend to swamp attention so people may find it hard to think of the downsides of drinking when faced with a drink, and find it hard to think of the upsides of drinking when they have a hangover.

A common component of MI is a decisional balance. Creating a decisional balance (i.e. considering good/not so good things about current and alternative behaviours) helps clients to pit benefits and costs against each other at once, so they can make a more rational and functional decision.

Balance sheets are best developed as collaborative activities, and are usually written on a sheet of paper or whiteboard. The client should be encouraged to take the more active role. If a whiteboard is used, hand the marker to the client. However, if practitioners become aware that a client is anxious about writing, they write the issues down themselves, using the client's own words. If clients have trouble reading, they use drawings.

Motivational interviewing is not about making lists or being more knowledgeable. Since decisions are about how we feel, and whether those feelings tip us towards change, MI practitioners probe emotional reactions to costs (e.g. 'does that concern you?') or may play devil's advocate ('but that hasn't really affected you much, has it?') in order to encourage clients to consider whether an impact is significant. In addition, since dysfunctional behaviour is typically inconsistent with core values (long life, not hurting others, being a good parent, etc.), practitioners may elicit those values and encourage the client to consider whether there are discrepancies between core values and current behaviours. This consideration tends to elicit discomfort and provides powerful motivation for change.

Motivational interviewing is informed by theories of change. MI has often been linked with Prochaska & DiClemente's (1982) transtheoretical model of change, which proposes that people typically pass through identifiable stages in the process of achieving lasting change.

- Precontemplation, when the person does not acknowledge the need for change.
- Contemplation, when the need for change is acknowledged but there is no resolution to achieve change.

- Determination or Preparation, when the person decides to make a change and develops concrete plans.
- Action, when change commences.
- Maintenance, when change is sustained.

If relapse occurs, the person may revert to one of the previous 'stages' or states in the cycle of change.

The transtheoretical model of change can be helpful in the application of motivational interviewing, because the focus of MI interventions will be different depending on the stage of change that the person is currently in. However, it is important to understand that change is not a simple linear process. People can move between stages quite fluidly. The practitioner needs to be alert to the person's current state of mind, rather than assuming that someone who was in contemplation last week will continue to be in contemplation or will have moved forward to determination.

Contemplation is the prototypical stage for using MI and helping the person decide what they want to do. However, MI can be used at any stage, although it changes its nature depending on where the person is in relation to the decision.

- In Precontemplation, people are typically happy to talk about the benefits of their current behaviour and may be tempted to admit to some downsides. They may also agree on a situation where they would consider the issue further (e.g. 'if I got a smoker's cough, I would probably think more seriously about it'). This gives the practitioner a context where they clearly have permission to return to the subject.
- If people are in Determination/Preparation, reviewing their key motivations for change, self-challenging beliefs about the costs of change, consolidating confidence and making detailed plans can help to move them to Action.
- In Action and Maintenance, the focus tends to be similar, except that new benefits of change emerge, current concerns about the costs of change may need to be addressed, and emerging problems need to be met with effective plans.
- If relapse occurs, the person may revert to Precontemplation or Contemplation thinking. However, there may be an additional problem of feeling disheartened about falling back into the old behaviour: major foci therefore are usually building confidence by highlighting (and praising) successes and helping the person solve problems they previously encountered.

Does motivational interviewing require the practitioner to endorse unhealthy lifestyles?

Practitioners are sometimes concerned that the focus of exploring client decision-making processes, and especially being willing to consider the benefits or advantages of inherently unhealthy activities such as smoking, might endorse or even encourage such behaviour.

Motivational interviewing requires a genuine interest in client motivations and an openness to learning about them. It also requires practitioners to accept that clients must take responsibility for their own lifestyle decisions and any consequences that occur. This does not mean that practitioners are endorsing these decisions either tacitly or explicitly.

How can MI help Sam with his smoking?

At the moment, Sam does not think he has made any decision about smoking. He is not even thinking about it most of the time. He would prefer not to think about it because if he does, he would have to acknowledge that it is costing him a lot of money and damaging his health. When people like his doctor force him to think about it, Sam's main aim is to extricate himself so he can avoid it. So, when his doctor last mentioned that he should quit smoking, Sam responded by saying 'I'll think about it'. What he actually meant was 'I won't think about it'.

Making the external internal

As noted above, a core aim of MI is to shift the change discourse from an argument between one person and another to a debate within the person.

Sam is pretty comfortable with the dialogue he has with his doctor. He has had a thousand such discussions before, starting in childhood with his mother. He does not enjoy them, but he knows what to do to escape. Most importantly, they don't make him want to quit. As far as he is concerned, they are just more nagging from people who think they know what is good for him – they don't understand how he feels about smoking, and it seems they don't want to know.

Sam is in 'Precontemplation' most of the time. Every now and then, especially when he is short of money, he thinks, 'I wish I could give up these damn things' and moves temporarily into Contemplation, but that is usually as far as it goes. Once he did try some action: at the recommendation of his doctor, he agreed to try nicotine patches. However, he discovered that it was not just the nicotine but something about the act of smoking that kept him going. He went back to smoking after a day or two.

Choices are often made after some kind of internal debate. This internal debate reflects our ambivalence. Once we make a decision, we tend to put the debate behind us because it hinders the execution of our decisions. Motivational interviewing reactivates that internal debate, which allows reconsideration of the decision.

In reading the example below, notice that Sam's practitioner does not volunteer information. In MI, information is offered sparingly in the interview, usually to validate and augment the impact of a concern Sam has or to answer a question. Occasionally, it may also be offered to gently correct a false belief. The emphasis is on information that Sam wants to have, and on his feelings about it. Other information may be offered via handouts or other resources Sam can choose to view, so that the practitioner can avoid lecturing Sam or dominating the conversation.

Instead of just telling Sam he must stop smoking, Sam's practitioner invites him to join her in being curious about his smoking. In particular, she asks about some things that Sam finds enjoyable or helpful about smoking. When introducing these questions, it is important that they do not carry any implicit criticism, only genuine curiosity and interest. The key purpose of these and later questions is to elicit ambivalence about smoking; in order to fully understand both sides of that ambivalence (and the potential blocks to change), it is necessary for her and Sam to understand his motivations to smoke.

'Is it OK to talk about smoking for a while?' (Sam reluctantly agrees.)
'What do you like most about smoking?'
Sam seems surprised by the question. No one has asked him that before. He thinks for a few
    seconds, and says:
'It helps me get through the day, when I'm bored. It gives me something to do.'
She asks him to write that down. She is sitting next to him, so they can both see what is being
    written.
'Any other good things about smoking?'
'It picks me up when I'm feeling down.'
'Anything else?'
'It gives me some energy, and helps me think more clearly, and get things done.'
'Any other good things about smoking?'
'A lot of other people who come here are smokers – it's good to sit outside with them and
    have a smoke.'
Sam or his practitioner summarises the left column of Sam's balance sheet (see Box 6.1).
'So, you said smoking helps you get through the day, it gives you something to do when you
    are bored and it picks you up when you are feeling down. You get more energy and think
    more clearly, and that helps you get things done. You also like being outside the centre with
    other smokers. Is that right?'
'That's about it.'
'Is there anything that you don't like as much about smoking?'
Sam pauses. 'It costs a lot.'
'It can be really expensive. How much does it cost you each week?' (This helps him to quan-
    tify the problem and explore its consequences.)
'About $100 a week.'
'So, that's $5200 a year. That is a lot. What would you do with that?' (Summing over a year,
    or 10 years, maximizes the emotional impact of the cost.)
'I'd have more fun, that's for sure. And maybe if I saved it, we could buy a better car.'
'Yes. Does that cost cause any problems for you?'
'It does mean we can't go out as much as I'd like. And Angela (his girlfriend) gives me
    heaps about it.'
'Does that upset you?' (Remember that motivation is mainly about emotions – tapping into
    the emotional connotations of downsides augments dissatisfaction.)
'Well, I certainly don't want to lose her.' (She suggests that he underline that, to show that it
    is very important to him.)

Rolling with resistance

Resistance to discussing behavior a person feels ambivalent about is natural and to be expected. Ambivalence is a state of internal conflict and is inherently uncomfortable. In motivational interviewing, the strategy is to 'roll with the resistance'. In other words, the practitioner does not 'push back' or try to overcome resistance with argument or other words of persuasion.

Clients may communicate overtly or covertly that they no longer want to discuss life-style change – at least at present. It is important not to press on in the face of this kind of

---

Box 6.1   Sam's smoking balance sheet

Good things about smoking	**Not so good things about smoking**
Helps me get through the day	Costs a lot ($5200 a year!)
Something to do	Can't go out much
Picks me up when I'm down	Angela is upset about the cost
Energy	Sometimes cough in the morning
Think more clearly	An addiction – I'm not in control
Get things done	
Enjoy being with other smokers	
I'm less grumpy with Angela	

Things I's miss if I stopped smoking	**Good things about stopping smoking**
Sitting with my friends outside the centre	Angela happier
Something to do	More money
	Breathe more easily
	Could have more fun
	Maybe could buy a better car?
	More in control

---

communication. It is much better to leave it to another day than to make it a point of contention between the client and the practitioner. Rolling with the resistance ensures that the argument remains an internal one and is not externalised into an unproductive argument between client and practitioner.

'Are there any other things that aren't so good about smoking?'
'I know it's bad for my health.' (If the practitioner did not pursue this, Sam may just be repeating what others have said. It is his concerns that will motivate him.)
'But what do you think?'
'I'm not sure.'
'Have you noticed any physical effects at all from smoking?' (She makes the issue concrete and checks for things that may be happening now; if there were nothing now, she would ask about any worries about his future health.)
'I do sometimes cough a bit in the morning but not all the time.'
'Yes, that is a common thing that happens with smoking. It's a sign that your lungs are reacting to the tar and other particles in the smoke. Does that worry you?' (Again, she looks for an emotional reaction.)
'Not really. It will go away if I stop smoking.'
'Yes, it probably will, and the long-term risks are much less as well.' (This is not a current concern, but she plants the seed for later discussion, if a concern emerges.)
'Anyhow, my grandfather smokes – he's in his 70s and he's OK.'
'You could be one of the lucky ones like your grandfather. Most smokers do get health complications but you might be an exception.' (This response avoids arguing with Sam and acknowledges that he could be right. But it also ensures he has information that the odds are not in his favour. It is then up to Sam what he does with that information.)
After checking for any more concerns, she summarises the things he does not like as much about smoking.
'So, you've noticed that you sometimes are coughing in the morning, but the thing that bothers you most about smoking is how much it costs, and the effects that cost is having. It is quite a sacrifice when you don't have a lot of money and sometimes you find you have to go without things you really need so that you can afford cigarettes – and it sounds like you are worried about Angela's reaction to that as well.'

Introducing the bigger picture: values and priorities

When people engage in unhealthy or self-destructive behaviour, they often dissociate this behaviour from their core values and/or long-term ambitions. This may occur because they have lost connection with these values or have come to feel that they have no prospect of achieving things they once felt to be important. Sometimes the values and ambitions remain alive but the incompatible behaviour is compartmentalised and kept separate from these values and ambitions.

The importance of core values and long-term life priorities is that they provide the compass that orients us in our life journey. People do not necessarily behave in accordance with values or priorities because there are all sorts of day-to-day exigencies and circumstances that take us off track. But as a general rule, people are happiest when on a path that is consistent with values and priorities. Going off the path creates a state termed cognitive dissonance which feels incongruent and wrong.

A strategy of MI is to activate underlying values and priorities and bring them into focus alongside the target behaviour. This means that it becomes clear to the client if he is off the path that is consistent with values and priorities and he experiences cognitive dissonance. It is often easier to change behaviour and get back on the path than to change values and priorities so as to make them consistent with the target behaviour. A conversation about values and priorities commonly therefore occurs in MI.

> Sam has already shared with his rehabilitation practitioner two core ambitions. He would like to be able to earn an income and support himself rather than relying on welfare. He would also like to have a family. He feels he could be a good father. Both these ambitions have been put on hold because of his experience of mental illness. He has become unsure whether he will ever be able to realise them.
>
> Sam's ambitions relate to his core values which can be summarised as:
>
> • self-reliance and autonomy
> • supporting others.

These values become relevant to MI when we invite Sam to align his smoking with these values. Being dependent on cigarettes is an affront to his core value of self-reliance and autonomy ('It's an addiction, I'm not in control'). The idea of being dependent creates cognitive dissonance and one way of resolving this is to show he is not dependent by taking steps to quit. Sam's value of support for others comes into play if we invite him to consider how his smoking affects other people.

> Sam says he knows he is not supporting Angela by spending so much money on cigarettes, but on the other hand, he might be more grumpy and difficult with Angela if he stopped smoking. He adds those to the list.

Learning about how unhealthy behaviour is sustained by core values such as a wish to protect a partner from irritable mood is just as important as learning how behaviour change can align with core values. In this case, Sam's rehabilitation worker realised that it might be important to involve Angela if Sam did decide to quit or even cut down on his smoking.

Sam's practitioner compares the lists on the top half of the sheet (see Box 6.1).
'So, which are most important to you?'
Sam says that his concern over Angela's reactions to his smoking and the cost of cigarettes are more important than the things he liked.

So Sam's practitioner asks what would change for the better if he stopped smoking. He says that he'd notice the extra money right away... and his girlfriend would be happier. When asked if there is anything else, he says he thinks he'd notice being able to breathe more easily.

His practitioner reminds him that he said the money would help him have more fun, and maybe even buy a car. He adds them to the list. She asks if it would help him feel more in control, and he adds that too.

She asks him if there was anything he would miss, and he says he'd miss sitting with his friends outside the centre. It would be too hard to sit there and not smoke.

She asks if it was always good, sitting there with them, and he replies that it wasn't always; in fact, it was often a bit boring (This is a form of brief cognitive therapy, checking if the beliefs about the good things are really as good as he thinks.)

She suggests that it may be important for them to work on finding other social outlets that didn't involve smoking, and were more fun. Sam agrees.

Notice that the balance sheet is not a static document. Often new benefits and costs will emerge as the client develops a clearer understanding of the behaviour, both in this and later sessions. For example, Sam did not initially identify the addictive quality of cigarettes as a disadvantage. It was only when invited to consider smoking in relation to the value he placed on autonomy that he realised that the addictive qualities of cigarettes really bothered him.

Sam's practitioner helps him to summarise the overall picture, and asks what he thinks about it. '*I guess I really do need to stop smoking. Only thing is, I don't think I can, so there's probably no point.*'

Building self-efficacy

Clients often lack confidence in being able to start behaviour change. Self-efficacy is not effectively built by reassurance. It is most effectively consolidated by reviewing past achievements (Box 6.2). These should be as close as possible to the task being considered, e.g. in this case, any quit-smoking attempts in the past, restriction of drinking or other substance use, dieting, exercise or other self-control behaviour.

Practitioners draw attention to achievements and successful strategies, and ask if any could be applied to the current attempt.

Box 6.2   Sam's self-efficacy sheet

0–100 confidence:	At start	At end
Things I've achieved before	How I did them	What I could do now (just put √ if the same)
Quit smoking for a week	Dad helped me take my mind off the cigarette	Angela could help me take my mind off it Nicotine patches

---

'OK, can we talk about your confidence for a bit? On a scale from 0–100, where 100 is being
   sure you can do it, how would you rate your confidence?'
'About 25%.'
'Have you ever tried to quit before?'
'Yes, I was hopeless. Only lasted a week.'
'Was that with nicotine patches?'
'No, couldn't afford them.'
'Then that's quite an achievement. You were probably almost through the worst of the nicotine
   withdrawal. How did you last that long?'
'I was living at home. My dad helped me take my mind off it when I wanted a smoke.'
'Now you're with Angela, could she help?'
'Yes, I guess so.'
'If I can help you get some patches for a few weeks, would that help as well?'
'Yes, that would be great.'

The list is continued. Sam's practitioner helps him list past achievements and strategies he
could use now. Then she asks him to re-rate his confidence – it is now 45. She draws Sam's
attention to the improvement, and tells him that that more detailed planning might help him
feel even more confident.

This is often a good place to stop the session and give clients the decisional balance and
self-efficacy sheets to take away, with a request that they read and add or delete ideas if
they wish. If you do this, make another appointment as soon as possible to see if Sam is
still wanting to make a change.

From decision to action?

After spending some time with his balance sheet and reflecting on what is important in his
life, Sam decides that he really does want to change his smoking behaviour. However, he is
not sure how to go about it. He does not now think he needs nicotine patches: 'It is not like
I am addicted to nicotine – I just like to smoke'. He is not sure he is ready to give up but he
would like to cut down on the amount he smokes, partly because it would save money and
partly because if he cuts down, it will show 'I am in control'.

If a client decides that they want to make a change, their practitioner helps them convert
their decision into action, by creating a plan.

Sometimes, clients do not choose an option that is likely to give them the outcomes they want (e.g. a reduction in alcohol consumption from 80 to 70 drinks per week). In MI, the practitioner will typically praise the determination that the client has to make a change, offer to help the client with the attempt, while also feeding back information about common issues that are faced by people adopting that goal (e.g. reducing drinking from 80 to 70 a week is difficult to accomplish and typically has only limited benefits). Together, they can keep track of how things go, and review the outcomes at an agreed time point.

Many smokers are like Sam, finding the idea of abrupt cessation a big step, whether or not nicotine replacement is present. A vague intention to reduce smoking tends to have poor outcomes (Cinciripini *et al.*, 1997). However, scheduled smoking reduction (progressively reducing the number of cigarettes over set periods) has shown positive results (Cinciripini *et al.*, 1997), as has reduction alongside gradually increased doses of nicotine replacement (Shiffman *et al.*, 2009). In both cases, a detailed plan is needed. Ultimately, the aim needs to be a reduction to zero, since there is no safe dose of inhaled tobacco smoke.

Before starting an attempt to change, it is important to obtain an accurate baseline. Methods to obtain assessments of daily behaviour, including self-monitoring and event-based recall (a 'Timeline Followback'), are described in Chapter 8.

> After feeding back this information, Sam's practitioner asks Sam what 'cutting down' means for him. Sam says he wants to halve his rate of smoking.
>
> Based on his purchases, Sam is currently smoking about 20 cigarettes a day. His practitioner suggests a more modest 20% reduction, to bring his smoking to 16 per day. She explains that this would mean having around one less cigarette over every 3 hours; for example, keeping four aside to have in each three-hour period, and waiting another 10–15 minutes before having each cigarette. She asks Sam if he thinks he could do that. Sam says 'yes'.

With any kind of behaviour change, it is better to overachieve than underachieve: setting small but meaningful targets is usually better than setting targets with high probability of failure. If Sam is able to beat 16 per day, that is fine. If he is unable to manage 16, it means that he is more dependent than he thought, and either a more modest goal or the addition of a small dose of nicotine replacement will be needed.

> Sam's practitioner notes that a 20% fall is different from the quit-smoking one they discussed in the last session, and asks him to rate it on the 0–100 scale; he gives it 90. He says that some of the same ideas would work; for example, Angela could help him take his mind off it. He'll also try to stay busy. Together, they start to make a plan (Box 6.3).

The role of the practitioner is that of consultant. Sam can decide how he wants to approach the challenge. The practitioner can use her knowledge and understanding of behaviour change principles to help him develop strategies with a reasonable chance of success. However, there is no single correct strategy and ultimately Sam will need to find out what works for him.

Box 6.3   Sam's plan to cut down his smoking

My overall goal
Cut smoking by 20% to ≤16 a day

How I'll do it
Put aside 4 cigarettes for each 3 hours
Delay each smoke for at least 10 minutes
Tell Angela
Buy one packet less for every 5 days

How confident I am
90% I can do it

When I'll need a plan
Tea/coffee time
When I'm bored
When I'm with smokers

What I'll do
Delay it for half an hour
Work on Angela's car
Talk to Angela to take my mind off it
Pace myself – make a cigarette last at least another 5 minutes

---

More detailed assessment shows that some of Sam's smoking occurs at predictable times (on waking, after meals, when drinking tea or coffee). He also smokes when he experiences a dysphoric mood he describes as boredom. His highest rate of smoking is when he is socialising with other smokers.

Some choices have to be made if he is to meet his 20% reduction target. For now, he wants to keep smoking with tea or coffee: he'll just delay when he has it (Later, it will be important to break this nexus, if he is to stop altogether.) Similarly, he doesn't want to stop socialising with other smokers altogether. He'll try to pace his smoking with them. When he reduces further or stops smoking altogether, he may need to cut down on the amount of time he spends with smokers, and spend more time with people who do not smoke. He may also need to develop ways to resist smoking, e.g. becoming adept at refusing cigarettes when offered.

Sam's practitioner asks whether he needs to make any preparations to get started. He says he'll tell Angela what he's trying to do, so she can help. Besides, he thinks she'll be really pleased he's making an effort. He'll also need to cut down the amount he buys, so he can keep track more easily; he'll stop buying cartons and make sure he buys a packet less for every five days. Already, he can see some savings!

Sam's practitioner suggests they make an appointment for the following week to see how he's going. Sam agrees.

Modifying motivational interviewing for schizophrenia

Cognitive problems often make it hard for people with psychoses to maintain attention, particularly when they try to hold multiple things in attention at once. These problems are likely to be especially evident when they are having an episode. Some changes from standard MI for the general population are often needed.

• If you notice the person's attention is wandering, remind them about the task. Consider taking a brief break or split MI over more than one session.

- Written or pictorial summaries are even more important than with other groups. Help them to rehearse what is on the summary sheet. Sometimes, a step needs to be repeated.
- Ask them to circle or underline one or two things on each side of a decisional balance sheet that are particularly important. Focusing on them reduces the cognitive load.
- Drawing a see-saw with 1–2 key elements on each side is sometimes needed, to help the person see what is most important to them.
- See if they would like any reminders to help them remember what they decided to do, e.g. a text message, wallet card or a sticker on each cigarette pack with the goal and coping strategies. See if there is a relative or friend they would like to help them remember (but check that this would not become intrusive).

Summary

Motivational interviewing is more than a set of strategies or steps, and it is more than making lists and plans. Those are just techniques that are commonly used to achieve the end. It is an empathic, client-centred approach that creates conditions where it is safe to talk about changing behaviour, where the client can be sure that they will not be bullied into change but can make their own decisions and have those decisions supported, whatever they are. These are attributes that make MI a style of interaction that can be used throughout rehabilitation, a style that involves listening more than talking, a style that accepts the person and helps them achieve what they value most.

References

Baker A, Turner A, Kay-Lambkin FJ, Lewin TJ (2009) The long and the short of treatments for alcohol or cannabis misuse among people with severe mental disorders. *Addictive Behavior* **34**, 852–8.

Banham L, Gilbody S (2010) Smoking cessation in severe mental illness: what works? *Addiction* **105**, 1176–89.

Cinciripini PM, Wetter DW, McClure JB (1997) Scheduled reduced smoking: effects on smoking abstinence and potential mechanisms of action. *Addictive Behaviors* **22**, 759–67.

De Hert M, Correll CU, Bobes J *et al.* (2011) Physical illness in patients with severe mental disorders. I. Prevalence, impact of medications and disparities in health care. *World Psychiatry* **10**, 52–77.

De Leon J, Diaz FJ (2005) A meta-analysis of worldwide studies demonstrates an association between schizophrenia and tobacco smoking behaviors. *Schizophrenia Research* **76**, 135–57.

Heckman CJ, Egleston BL, Hofmann MT (2010) Efficacy of motivational interviewing for smoking cessation: a systematic review and meta-analysis. *Tobacco Control* **19**, 410–16.

Hettema JE, Hendricks PS (2010) Motivational interviewing for smoking cessation: a meta-analytic review. *Journal of Consulting and Clinical Psychology* **78**, 868–84.

Kavanagh DJ, Mueser KT (2010) The treatment of substance misuse in people with serious mental disorders. In: Turkington D, Hagen R, Berge T, Gråwe RW (eds) *The CBT Treatment of Psychosis – A Symptomatic Approach*. Routledge: London, pp.161–74.

Kavanagh DJ, Young R, White A *et al.* (2004) A brief motivational intervention for substance abuse in recent-onset psychosis. *Drug and Alcohol Review* **23**, 151–5.

Lasser K, Boyd JW, Woolhandler S, Himmelstein DU, McCormick D, Bor DH (2000) Smoking and mental illness: a population-based prevalence study. *JAMA* **284**, 2606–10.

Miller WR, Baca LM (1983) Two-year follow-up of bibliotherapy and therapist-directed controlled drinking training for problem drinkers. *Behavior Therapy* **14**, 441–8.

Miller WR, Rollnick S (1991) *Motivational Interviewing: Preparing People to Change Addictive Behavior*. Guilford Press: New York.

Miller WR, Rollnick S (2002) *Motivational Interviewing: Preparing People for Change*, 2nd edn. Guilford Press: New York.

Prochaska JO, DiClemente CC (1982) Transtheoretical therapy: toward a more integrative model of change. *Psychotherapy: Theory, Research and Practice* **19**, 276–88.

Rogers CR (1959) A theory of therapy, personality, and interpersonal relationships as developed in the client-centered framework. In: Koch S (ed) *Psychology: The Study of a Science, vol. 3. Formulations of the Person and The Social Context*. McGraw-Hill: New York, pp.184–256.

Rollnick S, Miller W, Butler C (2008) *Motivational Interviewing in Health Care: Helping Patients Change*. Guilford Press: New York.

Shiffman S, Ferguson SG, Strahs KR (2009) Quitting by gradual smoking reduction using nicotine gum: a randomized controlled trial. *American Journal of Preventive Medicine* **36**, 96–104.

Ziedonis D, Hitsman B, Beckham J *et al*. (2008) Tobacco use and cessation in psychiatric disorders: National Institute of Mental Health Report. *Nicotine and Tobacco Research* **10**, 1–25.

Chapter 7

Individual Recovery Planning: Aligning Values, Strengths and Goals

Trevor Crowe, Frank P. Deane and Lindsay Oades

Sam is feeling a bit despondent. He is not depressed but he feels he does not know where he is heading in life. Working with his rehabilitation practitioner is helping with some specific challenges but he is feeling a bit lost in the bigger picture.

I know what I don't want, like I don't want to go back to hospital, I don't want to be broke or homeless. Who I want to be is all a bit vague to me though. I have tried setting goals for myself before, but when it comes down to making them happen I kind of lose motivation, I can't get my head together and just forget about what I promised myself to do. I find the rehab boring at times. Some of the activities are OK I guess. I go along because it is expected of me. I guess it helps but I just don't seem to be getting anywhere. I remember saying to one of the guys at the rehab that I wanted to go to university one day and get a degree and make something of myself. He laughed at me and said I was being unrealistic, that I can't even remember to take my medication so how could I get through a degree. I felt crushed. Perhaps he's right.

This chapter describes collaborative goal-setting steps and a protocol that is underpinned by goal-directed principles. It is important to recognise that goals have different sources of motivation and that a major strategy in our approach involves linking goals with underlying values and strengths to tap into those sources of motivation. As part of this process, we try to help the person shape a personal life vision. Thus, goal setting creates 'a concrete road map that mediates between where the person is and where he or she desires to go' (Ades, 2004, p.15). Whilst collaborative goal setting is important, the values underpinning the goal and the vision driving the goal are also very important. This chapter focuses particularly on helping the person with a mental illness clarify life values and a vision. This vision is a great source of motivation and is essential for identifying goals, particularly approach-oriented goals (i.e. goals moving towards something positive).

Goal setting is most effective when it occurs within a working relationship where the practitioner is sensitive to the client's readiness, motivations and orientation to his/her recovery process. There is often a need to socialise the client to goal setting and to build hope. Most clients come with needs-based goals that tend to be driven by an 'avoidance' motivation (i.e. to move away from or change an undesirable experience) and while these should be attended to, the aim is to help the client move toward growth-based goals that tend to have an 'approach' motivation.

Goal setting is a fundamental part of psychosocial rehabilitation and recovery support. The quality of goal setting is determined by:

* the authenticity of collaboration
* the degree to which the client 'owns' the goals
* the number of goal-directed principles used
* the effective balance of the meaning and manageability of goals
* how well specific goals are integrated with the action steps to attain the goals.

Clarke *et al.* (2009a) found that the goal attainment of people with enduring mental illness mediated the relationship between their ratings of symptom distress and their perception of personal recovery. That is, goals are central to the recovery process, particularly in relation to facilitating growth, empowerment and wellbeing. The steps outlined below are designed to operationalise the goal-setting principles.

Socialising the person to goal-setting processes

It is important to recognise from the start that people will have a range of reactions to goal setting that often include increased anxiety, refuting the value of goal setting, feeling that goal setting is a bit like a test or something they may be held accountable for, or not understanding what it means or involves. Therefore, an important part of 'authenticity in collaboration' is making sure the person is appropriately engaged and socialised to each of the steps along the way, including exploring and explaining how the collaborative relationship works. The aim here is to help the person understand that recovery involves taking appropriate risks and accepting that progress will feel uncomfortable at times. It is important to clarify with the client that they are the one who makes the decisions about what they want to work on and that the practitioner's role is to support the person in making the changes they want. Finally, the practitioner should reinforce that goal setting helps improve the chances of people moving forward in the desired directions (Box 7.1).

A care plan audit tool based on goal-setting theory and research evidence ('Goal-IQ', Goal Instrument for Quality) has been developed to assess the quality of goals being set in mental health services (Clarke *et al.*, 2009b). A revision called the Goal and Action Plan Instrument for Quality (GAP-IQ) incorporates the action-planning components of the goal-planning and -monitoring process and is displayed in Box 7.2. This is an audit tool and consists of 17 key goal quality and action-planning domains that provide a structured guide for practitioners when reviewing their care planning with clients. Reviewing each of the 17 items of the GAP-IQ provides a useful way to specify the various steps that should be considered when goal planning with clients.

Before engaging in the specific steps, it is important to have established rapport and a good working alliance with the client. This increases client engagement, collaboration and ownership of any plans and actions. This initial relationship development process also helps the practitioner identify motivation, prior success, strengths, confidence and

---

Box 7.1   Goal-directed principles

- The degree of goal agreement between the client and the practitioner is linked to increased satisfaction, decreased distress, reduced symptomatology and improved rehabilitation outcomes (Michalak *et al.*, 2004).
- The more the client is actively engaged in their own goal setting, the better their rehabilitation outcomes (Tryon & Winograd, 2001).
- Goal attainment is improved when meaning and manageability are optimised (Little, 1989).
- Goals are more manageable when they are not set too far into the future (Bandura & Simon, 1977) and when the client is at least 70% confident that they could achieve the goal within a set time period (Clarke *et al.*, 2006).
- Ensuring that goals are in line with the client's values, interests, dreams and preferred identity is likely to increase goal ownership and in turn goal attainment (Anthony, 1991; Clarke *et al.*, 2006, 2009; Sheldon & Houser-Marko, 2001).
- Goal quality is defined by the degree to which goals are:
  - clearly defined
  - measurable
  - sufficiently difficult/challenging to be engaging without being overwhelming
  - integrated with an action plan
  - time framed
  - monitored for goal progress
  - inclusive of progress feedback and problem solving of barriers (Locke & Latham, 1990).

---

other resources that will help the person move forward with their goals. If the practitioner imposes goal setting on the person before they are ready to explore goal options, it is likely to be met with resistance. Strategies to operationalise these principles are elaborated on in Box 7.2.

In Chapter 6 some of the aims and techniques of motivational interviewing were described. Of particular relevance to goal setting are the issues of 'what the person is ready for' and how the conversations regarding goal setting can be 'shaped' to maximise ownership, engagement and consequently readiness. It is important to bear in mind that if the person is feeling overwhelmed with unmet needs, they may seem less ready to talk about goals but rather be concerned only with seeking some relief and safety. However, meeting unmet needs does usually involve goal setting. The goals that target unmet needs tend to be quite immediate in focus and more about getting away from an undesirable experience (i.e. avoidance-oriented goals) than about moving towards a preferred life direction (i.e. approach-oriented goals). Avoidance- and approach-oriented goals tend to have different sources of motivation. The practitioner therefore needs to be aware of how to work with these different motivational sources. Avoidance-oriented goals are more about problem clarification and problem solving/management, while approach goals are about clarifying what is important to the person (i.e. what they value) and what they want to move towards. Approach goals involve helping the person shape their life vision and pursuing goals that represent the person's vision for themselves. Approach goals can be distinguished from avoidance goals by reflecting on whether the motivation is primarily to relieve a current situation or to move toward a more positive situation.

Box 7.2 Goal and Action Plan Instrument for Quality (GAP-IQ)

1. Is there an overall recovery vision?	No	No written record to indicate that any of the following were discussed with the client: meaning, hopes, dreams, values and/or preferred identity that the person wishes to head towards or practise in their life
	Partial	Written record that hopes, dreams and values for the future have been discussed but the goals selected do not appear to be in line with the client's values or there is no record that the client has been asked why they would like to achieve their set goals
	Yes	Written record that hopes, dreams and values for the future have been discussed. There is a direct link between the meaning, hopes and dreams that the individual holds for their future and goals selected within case management and these are documented (e.g. 'Client reported that doing his own shopping (goal) would lead him to feel more independent (recovery vision)')
2. Collaboration between client and practitioner	No	Language in the care plan does not suggest that collaboration between client and practitioner occurred when identifying care plan goals (e.g. 'client was instructed to work on medication adherence', 'client was provided with goals set out by his mental health team'). Or there is language in the file that describes the client or their goals in negative terms (e.g. lacks insight, unrealistic, unmotivated)
	Yes	Language in the care plan indicated that collaboration between practitioner and client occurred when developing goals. Goals are recorded in layperson's terms void of technical jargon
3. Goals	No	No goals are recorded
	Partial	Some goals are recorded yet they are not clearly defined, making measurement difficult (e.g. to feel better, to be happier)
	Yes	Goals are recorded and defined so that a clear outcome is measurable (e.g. to do my own shopping, improve my medication taking, find a job)
4. Goal importance	No	No record that the client's perceived importance of goals selected or prioritisation of the care plan goals was determined
	Partial	A written record that the client's perceived importance for each goal has been considered and resources allocated accordingly (e.g. 'client stated that ___ goal was most important for them, so the session was spent working toward this')
	Yes	A record that goal importance has been ranked numerically or ordered and resources allocated accordingly (e.g. 'client placed goals in order of importance (1, 2, 3) so session time and tasks were allocated with this in mind')
5. Confidence	No	No written record that the client's level of confidence was rated for the goals selected
	Partial	Written record that confidence was asked (e.g. a statement or rating) in relation to one of the goals but not others. A written record that client confidence was assessed, yet goals were not adjusted to enhance the client's self-efficacy related to goal attainment
	Yes	A written record that confidence was determined in relation to each case management goal and goals were adjusted to enhance the client's confidence for goals attainment

6. Timeframe for goals	No	No timeframe established for goals achievement
	Partial	Some record of a timeframe for goal completion but this is vague (e.g. end of the year, rather than a specific date). Or the timeframe seems unrealistic for the type of goal selected (e.g. to commence and complete a TAFE course within 3 months)
	Yes	Written record of an established timeframe and a date set for the review period
7. Levels of goal attainment	No	No varying levels of goal attainment defined for the treatment goals recorded
	Partial	Some but not all the case management goals have different levels of goal attainment defined and recorded. Levels for goals are defined but they are not behaviourally defined, making outcome difficult to measure (e.g. lacks specifications such as frequency, what, where and with whom)
	Yes	Attainment Levels for each of the case management goals are specified and behaviourally defined (e.g. frequency, what, where, with whom) so outcome can be clearly measured
8. Identifying and solving barriers to goal attainment (coping planning)	No	No written record that barriers to goal attainment are identified in the care plan. Or, if no barriers are described, there is also no evidence that potential barriers were discussed and solutions to address these identified
	Partial	A written record that some potential barriers were discussed but no problem solving around these is evident (e.g. lack of money may be a problem yet attempts to assist budgeting or identify alternative solutions are not evident). Only some of the treatment goals were recorded as being the focus of coping planning
	Yes	A written record that barriers and potential solutions for each of the treatment goals have been discussed
9. Social support	No	No written record that social support was enlisted to assist with goal attainment
	Partial	Written record that some social support was identified, either only at a service level (case manager) or personal level (family member)
	Yes	Written record that social support was discussed and identified to assist with goal attainment, at both a personal and service level. Roles for different members have been discussed and outlined. This can include practical (e.g. transportation), emotional (e.g. to hear the person's concerns) or informational support (e.g. information on harm minimisation or side-effects of medication, etc.)
10. Monitoring	No	No written record regarding how goal progress will be monitored
	Partial	General written reference made to monitoring progress (e.g. 'will check progress with client')
	Yes	Specific written record of how progress of behaviours in specific settings will be monitored (e.g. 'in addition to homework tasks, client has agreed to keep a graph of his number of walks or a mood diary')

11. Action plans for goals (general rating)	No	No record that discussions about pathways or strategies for any of the goals have taken place (e.g. steps to the goals)
	Partial	A written record that some of the case management goals have plans outlining how the goal will be achieved. Or a written record that the treatment goals have plans developed, yet these are not defined or specified clearly
	Yes	A written record that all goals selected have clear pathways of how to attain the goal and the specific details about when, where and how the goal will be carried out. Target goal must be specified in action plan
12. Action *Description*	No	Not completed
	Partial	Item attempted but insufficient or inappropriate information
	Yes	Item completed well. The task should be described in sufficient detail that the client and practitioner have a clear understanding of what the task is
13. Action *How often* specified	No	Not completed or inappropriate (e.g. run in the park)
	Partial	Item attempted but insufficient or inappropriate information. Description is not specific but an attempt has been made to record a response (e.g. 'as required', 'when I feel like it')
	Yes	Item completed well. Clearly describes the number of times the task should be completed (e.g. numeric 2 times, each morning, daily)
14. Action *When* specified	No	Not completed or inappropriate response (e.g. run in the park)
	Partial	Item attempted but insufficient or inappropriate information. Description is not specific but an attempt has been made to record a response (e.g. 'when required, when I feel in the mood, when I think about it')
	Yes	Item completed well. Clearly describes the time and/or date that the specific task is to be completed (e.g. morning, afternoon, night; 12pm, 3am, etc.; Monday, Tuesday, etc.; each morning before breakfast)
15. Action *Where* specified	No	Not completed or clearly inappropriate (e.g. run every morning). Where the task should be completed
	Partial	Item attempted but insufficient. Description is not specific (e.g. Wherever I get a chance)
	Yes	Item completed well. Clearly describes where the task should be completed. Specific location (e.g., home, around the block, at the hospital).
16. Action *Confidence* rating	No	Not completed. No confidence rating provided
	Partial	The confidence scale has a number circled that is less than 70
	Yes	The confidence scale has a number greater than or equal to 70 circled
17. Action plan *Review*	No	Not completed. Neither a rating nor comment is provided to indicate that a review was conducted
	Partial	There was either a comment made or a formal rating, but not both.
	Yes	Item completed well. There is a formal rating of the quantity or quality of task completion made by either the client or mental health practitioner. There is a comment indicating that a review was conducted

An exclusive focus on avoidance goals is problematic. Pursuing more avoidance goals is related to less satisfaction and more negative feelings about progress with personal goals; decreased levels of self-esteem, personal control and vitality, and less life satisfaction and feelings of competence (Elliot *et al.*, 1997).

Assisting the person to identify strengths is important regardless of whether they are currently focused on pursuing goals to meet unmet needs (i.e. to overcome or manage problems) or whether they are looking for ways to step forward to enact and embody their life vision. Clarifying strengths (i.e. what the person can rely on to feel stronger/ more confident, what keeps them strong) is about 'consolidating' where one is up to, catching one's breath and finding resources to draw on to move forward through the next challenge.

Sam's attempts at identifying values

At the beginning of the chapter, we noted that Sam was struggling to find a direction in life. As Sam's rehabilitation practitioner, how can you help him? There are several key issues in Sam's story that have direct implications for goal setting.

- How ready is Sam to set goals?
- What type of goals is Sam thinking about?
- How can the practitioner increase Sam's engagement and ownership of his goals?
- What is meaningful or important for Sam, and how can the practitioner retain that meaningfulness while helping Sam set manageable goals?
- How can the practitioner help Sam to clarify his recovery/life vision? That is, how can the practitioner help Sam to shape his 'preferred identity' and clarify the person he wants to be and the life he wants to live?
- What strengths does Sam already have, upon which his recovery can be built? How can the practitioner help Sam to build further strengths and increase his confidence to move forward in his recovery?
- How to manage memory and concentration issues as part of the goal-setting process?
- How can the practitioner develop a working alliance to help Sam to increase the likelihood of progressing with his goals?

Building strength

Recovery is built on strengths, not weaknesses or problems. '… one cannot build on weakness. To achieve results, one has to use all available strengths … These strengths are the true opportunities' (Drucker, 1967, cited in Linley & Harrington, 2006).

It is very easy for mental health work to become focused exclusively on identifying and managing problems. Problems or weaknesses no doubt can be destabilising and represent 'what is wrong', whereas a strengths approach focuses on 'what is strong'. A problem focus is important, particularly in the early stages of recovery, but if this is all that is attended to, it can be discouraging and deplete confidence. A strengths focus aims to build confidence, hope and self-efficacy, which in turn positively affect wellbeing. There should be an equivalent focus on identifying and building on existing strengths, as well as pursuing goals aimed at developing further strength.

It is helpful to have a broad view of what constitutes a strength, rather than just seeing it as talents or things that the person is good at. Strengths can also be resources, skills, beliefs, relationships, values that have been enacted, and memories that the person can call upon to support them through challenging situations, and in the pursuit of goals. Strengths also help build resilience, the capacity to bounce back from setbacks and push through obstacles. As recovery is not just about achieving some control of problems but also features many obstacles, setbacks and risks, it is very important that the person can access as much strength as possible to consolidate gains and push forward. Examples of practical strengths assessments are discussed elsewhere in this book (see Chapter 4).

Clarifying values and valued life directions

Recovery is about living a life that has personal meaning, purpose and fulfilment. Values clarification involves the person taking a step back from everyday life for a moment to focus on what is important to them and to start to map out the direction(s) in which they want to go. Values are linked to one's vision of one's preferred life and developing identity. However, values are accessible moment to moment regardless of whether one lives them out or not, or whether they seem to point to longer term goals. Exploring values can help strengthen the collaborative relationship between the client and practitioner as well as helping clients to:

- take stock in terms of identifying where they are living their lives in line with the things that are important to them, and where they are not
- identify where there may be conflicts between values being enacted and those that are suppressed as a result
- activate emotions and subsequent motivation to make changes in their lives
- shape the identity that reflects these values.

There are numerous ways of defining values. Some models consider values as principles of life, virtues or life directions (Linley & Harrington, 2006; Peterson & Seligman, 2004). However, put more simply, values are the things that are important to the person. Sometimes the process of 'valuing' is emphasised to suggest that values are not just something a person holds but something they do or could be enacting more. When values have been enacted, they can also then be considered strengths because these experiences can be drawn upon to access confidence and conviction to move further in these preferred life directions.

At times, reflecting on personal values can evoke an awareness of important neglected parts of one's life. For example, a person may realise that he really values creativity but has spent no time in the last couple of years expressing his creativity. This doesn't mean the person values creativity any less, just that enactment of this value has decreased, perhaps because he has been spending considerable time enacting other values (e.g. working or improving health) or that he has perhaps been letting certain barriers or obstacles get in his way. At times, people can become quite emotional when they review their lives, particularly in terms of how much they are currently living out their values.

This emotion can be redirected into pursuing goals and actions that support preferred changes in the enactment of these values.

Values have been described as 'global life directions' (Hayes, 2004) in that they reflect who the person wants to be and how they want to relate to the world. Values cannot be 'completed' *per se*; they are ongoing ways of living (Peterson & Seligman, 2004). For example, a client may value being a loving brother. This is an ongoing pursuit which may fluctuate in priority at different times during his life, but is never 'given up' or 'completed'. In contrast, good goal definition is such that there is a clear completion point within a predetermined timeframe. From our example, a goal in pursuit of the value 'being a loving brother' may be 'to visit my sister once a month over the next 3 months'.

It is important to find ways of exploring values (i.e. what is important to the person) that make sense to the client. Just asking 'what are your values?' will probably be met with blank stares or confusion. General questions such as the following often help people identify values or important life directions.

- What are the most important aspects of your life?
- What do you want your life to be about?
- What principles do you, or would you like to, live your life by?
- If you were to reveal your deepest longings for your life, what would they be?
- Imagining that there was no one to judge you, what would you most want for your life?
- What do you stand for?

More specific questions can be posed for particular life domains, as outlined in Box 7.3.

Sometimes using values or principles cards can be helpful in getting the person to think about things that are most important to them (for example, see Ciarrochi & Bailey,

---

Box 7.3 Questions to help clarify values in specific domains

If the person is having difficulty connecting with their values, the following questions may assist with some common values domains.

Work/education: What do you value in your work? What would make it more meaningful? What personal qualities would you like to bring to your work? What sort of relationships would you like to build with your work colleagues? What do you value about learning/education/training? What new skills would you like to learn? What knowledge would you like to gain?

Leisure: What sort of sports, leisure activities or hobbies do you enjoy? What do you find fun? How do you relax after a hard day? What is it that you enjoy most about these activities?

Relationships: What personal qualities would you like to bring to your relationships with family members/friendships and other intimate people? What sort of relationships would you like to build? How would you prefer to interact in these relationships? What is most important to you in the way you relate to others?

Personal growth/health: How do you want to look after your health – physical, mental, emotional and spiritual? Why is this important to you? What is most important to you in the area of spirituality (this may be a formal religion or as simple as connecting with nature)? If you were looking after yourself in the way that you wished, what would you be doing? What would that look like? How would you like to contribute to your community?

Box 7.4   Summary of values clarification

1. **Why clarify values?**
   a) There are benefits to wellbeing of having a clear sense of what one values.
   b) Goals change but values tend to stay the same. Values can provide meaning in day-to-day life.
   c) Clarifying values helps people to focus on what is important to them in life.
2. **What values are important to the person?**
   a) Values can vary from person to person.
   b) Help the person identify values using suggested strategies and questions above.
   c) Get the person to write down these values.
   d) Identify and list some strengths they would like to develop further.
3. **How well is the person living in alignment with their values?**
   a) Get the person to describe or rate how much they believe they have put each of these values into action within the past month. Questions such as 'Can you think of examples of when you have been enacting this value in your life over the last month?' can be helpful.
   b) Explore and discuss how well actions have been in alignment with values for the last month. This may involve an exploration of: (1) any feelings that arise, (2) any conflicts between different values (e.g. working a lot at the cost of time with family), (3) what strengths they see, and (4) what they want to do about adjusting the enactment of these values in their lives.
4. **How can the person use this to develop their life vision?**
   Ask the person to think of a life in which they live their values. That is, they think and act each day in a way that helps them live more consistently with their valued directions in life. This is also a way to help the person clarify their preferred identity, and provides a challenge for them to step up and start 'being this person'.

2008). Similarly, we use the metaphor of a recovery or life 'journey' which is readily identified and accepted by many clients with severe mental illness. We have also developed a series of 'tools' that are linked to this metaphor which support the process of identifying values and other aspects of goal planning and monitoring (see Oades & Crowe, 2008).

Align goals with valued life directions

After valued life directions have been clarified (Box 7.4), it is important to identify and align goals with these directions. Again, we have developed templates as part of the LifeJET protocols to facilitate this process (Oades & Crowe, 2008), but the following steps capture this process.

- Ask the person to choose up to three valued life directions to work on over the next 3 months or so. Doing so ensures that the goals are personally meaningful and in line with the person they want to be. Write down these valued directions so they are explicit and directly connected to goals that are to be developed. Some people decide to work on just one valued life direction at a time and set a series of goals related to it to increase activities that demonstrate that they choose to live their lives more in line with that valued life direction.

- Identify a specific goal for each of the valued directions. Try and select target goals that could be achieved in the next few months. Try to get the person to break down any longer-term goals into smaller steps.

Specify target goals

Write down up to three target goals. The target goals should be:

- specific and clearly defined, as shown in Sam's example
- challenging but something that the client is at least 70% confident of achieving in the decided timeframe
- able to be measured in terms of progress (i.e. you will know when you get there).

Resist the temptation to have more than one thing listed within each of the target goals (e.g. to go to a yoga class and walk for 10 km each week). It can deplete motivation and makes it more difficult to accurately review progress and overcome barriers if the person is only able to achieve part of what they have listed. It is better to make these separate goals for the same valued life direction. If the person is more than 85% confident that they will achieve their target goal in the allotted timeframe, it may not be a big enough step to be taking at this stage. Interestingly, people tend to be less motivated to pursue goals that are not challenging enough (i.e. they are highly confident that they will easily achieve them) or are too difficult (i.e. they lack sufficient confidence) (Locke *et al.*, 1981).

Identify levels of success

Sometimes when working towards goals, people achieve more than expected and sometimes, for many different reasons, they may not quite achieve all they had hoped. Writing down the 'levels of success' or 'levels of attainment' is helpful for both clients and mental health practitioners in tracking progress towards goals.

- For each target goal, get the person to write something that they might achieve that would be *better* than expected in the next few months. That is, the person is less confident that they would be able to achieve this in the timeframe set, and would see this as a real bonus if they were able to achieve this.
- For each target goal, get the person to write something that would be *less* than what they hoped to achieve in the next few months. That is, it may not be much more than what they are already achieving, and they would be disappointed if that was all they achieved in the allotted timeframe.

Review the goal plan

Set a time for when the goal is to be achieved. This will be the time set aside to review progress. It would be beneficial for a support person to know about the goals and to discuss progress (Box 7.5).

Box 7.5   Example: part of Sam's goal plan

My life vision is: to be true to myself, honest and respectful, never giving up

	Valued direction A To pursue knowledge
Higher level goal	To be enrolled in a course of my choice
Target goal *(Confidence 70%)*	Meet with course advisor at further education college by October 30th
Lower level goal	Review overviews of courses available for next year
Review details	I will review my progress with these goals on the following date: Monday November 5th I will share my goals and discuss progress with them with: my friend Bob

---

Collaborative action planning and monitoring

Action planning or therapeutic homework, as it is more commonly referred to in research publications, is known to improve outcomes for people with a range of clinical conditions (Kazantzis *et al.*, 2000; Kelly *et al.*, 2006). Furthermore, the degree of systematic implementation of action plans is linked to better treatment outcomes (Kelly & Deane, 2009). The steps for systematic action planning have been elaborated previously and are summarised below. However, the use of standard forms to structure and document this process is recommended (see Kelly & Deane, 2009, for examples).

The pathway to a goal is made up of a number of small action steps. Deciding what actions are required to attain goals is 'action planning'. Important steps in action planning are outlined in the GAP-IQ (particularly from point 8 onwards) (see Box 7.2).

The LifeJET protocols that we have developed provide a structure to support these important components of action planning and provide a written record for the client and the mental health practitioner. It is important that the client takes a written copy of the action plan away with them following a meeting in order to remind themselves of the specifics of the task and as a cue to take action. As with other parts of goal planning, it is essential that the client is actively and collaboratively involved in developing their action plan. Ownership of the action plan can be reinforced further by having the client write out the various details of the plan wherever possible.

The following steps for action planning are recommended; depending on the specifics of the behaviours, some components may not be necessary (e.g. length of time to engage in a particular behaviour may be as long as is needed for a specific task).

Action planning steps

1. Write the value and target goal at the top of the form.
2. Write the action that is required and elaborate on what this specifically entails.
3. Document the date the action was set, how often, when and where the person plans to engage in this action. Note that some 'actions' will be required only once. For example, 'telephone the local studio to enquire about yoga times', whilst others will be ongoing, 'go to yoga once a week on a Saturday morning'.
4. Write down any support required. The person will not always require all types of support for each action, but it is good practice to identify at least one person who can provide the client with emotional encouragement and support.
5. Document how the person intends to remind themselves of their commitment.
6. Brainstorm possible barriers they may encounter. This helps the person plan for the unexpected as much as possible. Barriers may be internal (such as thoughts and emotions) or external (for example, finances, time barriers, factors in the environment like bad weather preventing a picnic).
7. Brainstorm ways of addressing possible barriers.
8. Get the person to rate their confidence in completing the specific action from 0 to 100. As a guide, we suggest that the person choose something that they are fairly confident that they will achieve (confidence rating should be at least 70 out of 100). Ensure the action is not too easy or the person will be less likely to feel the satisfaction of achievement, but not so hard that they become frustrated and disappointed.
9. Set a review date for the action. Be sure to review progress at the next meeting. Encourage and reinforce achievements.
10. Accountability. The client should identify someone to tell about this plan so that they can encourage and support them, and this should be noted.

Summary

Goal setting is common practice in mental health settings. However, how well this is done is highly variable. The more that good goal-setting principles and practices are used when helping the individual to develop a recovery plan, the more likely that progress will be made toward goals. Recording the results of recovery planning conversations is recommended for the purposes of having a concrete record to direct and track progress, assisting with memory cuing, identifying strengths, values, goals and actions, and consolidating the person's life vision. Considering the person's readiness to engage in various aspects of recovery planning is an important part of engaging and socialising them to strategies that may help them move forward, and encouraging ownership of the recovery plan.

Ownership and personal meaning of the recovery plan are increased if values clarification is an integrated part of goal setting and action planning. Using a 'strengths' approach throughout the recovery planning process (including during the review of goal and action plan progress) helps build confidence, capacity and wellbeing, which in turn increases the likelihood of the person persisting through challenges and barriers to their recovery aspirations.

References

Ades A (2003) Mapping the journey: goal setting. *Psychosocial Rehabilitation* **5**, 1–75.

Anthony WA (1991) Recovery from mental illness: the new vision of services researchers. *Innovations and Research* **1**, 13–14.

Bandura A, Simon K (1977) The role of proximal intentions in self-regulation of refractory behaviour. *Cognitive Therapy and Research* **1**, 177–93.

Ciarrochi J, Bailey A (2008) *A CBT Practitioner's Guide to ACT: How to Bridge the Gap Between Cognitive Behavioral Therapy and Acceptance and Commitment Therapy*. New Harbinger Publications: Oakland, CA.

Clarke SP, Oades LG, Crowe TP, Deane FP (2006) Collaborative goal technology: theory and practice. *Psychiatric Rehabilitation Journal* **30**, 129–36.

Clarke SP, Oades L, Crowe T, Caputi P, Deane FP (2009a) The role of symptom distress and goal attainment in assisting the psychological recovery in clients with enduring mental illness. *Journal of Mental Health* **18**, 389–97.

Clarke SP, Crowe T, Oades L, Deane FP (2009b) Do goal setting interventions improve the quality of goals in mental health services? *Psychiatric Rehabilitation Journal* **32**(4), 292–9.

Elliot AJ, Sheldon KM, Church MA (1997) Avoidance personal goals and subjective well-being. *Personality and Social Psychology Bulletin* **23**, 915–27.

Hayes SC (2004) Acceptance and commitment therapy, relational frame theory, and the third wave of behavioural and cognitive therapies. *Behaviour Therapy* **35**(4), 639–65.

Kazantzis N, Deane FP, Ronan K (2000) Homework assignments in cognitive and behavioral therapy: a meta-analysis. *Clinical Psychology: Science & Practice* **7**, 189–202.

Kelly PJ, Deane FP (2009) The relationship between therapeutic homework and clinical outcomes for individuals with severe mental illness. *Australian and New Zealand Journal of Psychiatry* **43**, 968–75.

Kelly PJ, Deane FP, Kazantzis N, Crowe TP, Oades LG (2006) Use of homework by mental health case-managers in the rehabilitation of persistent and recurring psychiatric disability. *Journal of Mental Health* **15**, 1–7.

Linley PA, Harrington S (2006) Strengths coaching: a potential-guided approach to coaching psychology. *International Coaching Psychology Review* **1**(1), 37–46.

Little BR (1989) Personal projects analysis: trivial pursuits, magnificent obsessions, and the search for coherence. In: Buss DM, Cantor N (eds) *Personality Psychology: Recent Trends and Emerging Directions*. Springer-Verlag: New York.

Locke EA, Latham, GP (1990) *A Theory of Goal Setting and Task Performance*. Prentice-Hall: Englewood Cliffs, New Jersey.

Locke EA, Shaw KN, Saari LM, Latham GP (1981) Goal setting and task performance: 1968–1990. *Psychological Bulletin* **90**, 125–52.

Michalak J, Klappheck MA, Kosfelder J (2004) Personal goals of psychotherapy patients: the intensity and the 'why' of goal-motivated behavior and their implications for the therapeutic process. *Psychotherapy Research* **14**, 193–209.

Oades LG, Crowe TP (2008) *Life Journey Enhancement Tools (Life JET)*. Illawarra Institute for Mental Health, University of Wollongong: Wollongong, NSW, Australia.

Peterson C, Seligman MEP (2004) *Character Strengths and Virtues: A Handbook and Classification*. Oxford University Press: New York.

Sheldon KM, Houser-Marko L (2001) Self-concordance, goal attainment, and the pursuit of happiness: Can there be an upward spiral? *Journal of Personality and Social Psychology* **80**, 152–65.

Tryon GS, Winograd G (2001) Goal consensus and collaboration. *Psychotherapy* **38**, 385–9.

Chapter 8

Activation and Related Interventions

Robert King and David J. Kavanagh

Sam is feeling down. Even though, by objective standards, he has made real progress in management of his illness and has been stable for more than 6 months, he is increasingly aware that he is likely to be taking medication for the rest of his life and that achieving things that other people take for granted is a struggle. At times he feels hopeless and even suicidal. Most of the time he just feels lacking in energy or enthusiasm. While he is relieved that his voices are not tormenting him, their absence makes him feel empty and alone. He is spending more time just lying on his bed because there is nothing he feels like doing. His girlfriend, Angela, is worried about him and Sam is sure that pretty soon she will get tired of him and leave. Whether his state could be described as a clinical depression is a moot point. Sam's psychiatrist has explained that people with a diagnosis of schizophrenia can experience episodes of depression like anyone else and has commenced a trial of antidepressant medication. However, there has not been much benefit after 6 weeks and Sam resents the medication as 'just one more drug I have to take'.

This is a challenging time for Sam's rehabilitation practitioner. Sam has always needed a certain amount of motivating but it seems different this time. He really does seem depressed.

Depression is common among people with a diagnosis of schizophrenia and may affect as many as 50% of people like Sam (Buckley *et al.*, 2009). There is surprisingly little known about treatment of depression in the context of schizophrenia (Whitehead *et al.*, 2003). While there was early optimism that atypical antipsychotics would reduce the prevalence of depression, there is little evidence that this has been the case and clinical trials have been inconclusive (Furtado & Srihari, 2008). While it is common practice to add antidepressant medication to the treatment regime when there is evidence of depression, it is unclear how effective this is (Whitehead *et al.*, 2003).

In this chapter, we will show how Sam's rehabilitation practitioner can use behavioural activation (Dimidjian *et al.*, 2011) to help Sam overcome his depression. Behavioural activation (BA) is a simple structured treatment for depression that has a good track record for effectiveness in the treatment of major depression (Sturmey, 2009; Cuijpers *et al.*, 2007). BA is well suited to treatment of people with impaired cognition because, unlike most psychotherapies, it does not rely on a person being able to use reasoning to

Manual of Psychosocial Rehabilitation, First Edition. Edited by Robert King, Chris Lloyd, Tom Meehan, Frank P. Deane and David J. Kavanagh.
© 2012 Blackwell Publishing Ltd. Published 2012 by Blackwell Publishing Ltd.

overcome depression. While there has been limited research into the effectiveness of BA with people who have a diagnosis of schizophrenia, a small open trial with this population in the UK (Mairs *et al.*, 2011) found that it was well received and was very effective in reducing both depression and negative symptoms.

Behavioural activation is also conceptually and practically uncomplicated for the practitioner. It is likely that for some practitioners, the programme outlined in this chapter will seem like a more thorough and systematic version of interventions they already use with depressed clients. A detailed manual (Lejuez *et al.*, 2011) is readily available and the programme in this chapter is partly based on the manual, partly on modifications recommended by Mairs *et al.* (2011) and partly on the experience of the authors using BA and related interventions in rehabilitation practice with people like Sam.

There are some differences between using BA in schizophrenia and using it with someone who has an uncomplicated depression. Readers who are already familiar with BA will notice that we suggest the introduction of some enjoyable activities and tasks *before* values and goals are considered. Small changes in activity, with associated improvements in mood, will help to show the client how worthwhile the lifestyle changes can be. However, the standard linkage to values and goals then allows for more long-term, sustained changes to occur.

While the changes to Sam at the moment do look different from how he was in the past, it may not just be the depression that is reducing activity.

- Check his medication. Antipsychotic medication should be at the minimum effective dose to avoid excessive sedation. Has the medication changed recently? Heavy doses will make it harder for Sam to become more active.
- The schizophrenia may also be reducing motivation to engage in activities, and the degree to which this occurs can change over time. Even simple activities (e.g. going for a 10-minute walk each day) can be difficult. In each session, you may need to help Sam review the benefits of making an effort, and the degree of change may often need to be gradual, to maximise the chance of completion. If some activities can be with a friend or relative, that may increase the chance that they occur.

Cognitive difficulties can make it more difficult for people like Sam to remember to do the activity, and why. We have made changes to standard instructions for BA in the description below, to take account of these potential difficulties. Depending on the time available for sessions and the cognitive abilities of the person, one step may often need to be split or repeated over more than one session if the person is having difficulty concentrating. At regular points in each session, check that the client understands and can recall the content, e.g. ask them to summarise what you have both been discussing. If they show attentional or memory lapses, see if you can take a break for a few minutes or delay further work until your next contact. When you return to the discussion, give them a brief summary and check they understand, before moving on.

Introducing behavioural activation

While BA is simple, it will make demands on Sam and it is important he understands what he has to do and why you are asking him to do these things.

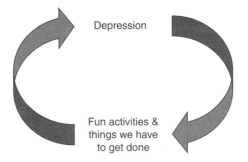

Figure 8.1   Relationship between depression and activity.

Sam may already know that he is feeling different from usual and is depressed. However, sometimes people just slip into depression and it feels as if it is their normal state. When this happens, it is important the person becomes aware that how he is feeling now is not how he usually feels. This can often be done by pointing to levels of activity and interest in the recent past. For example, 'You always used to watch football on television but now you can't be bothered' or 'You used to play your guitar most days but you haven't done that for 2 months'. A family member, partner or friend can often help identify changes in interests or activities.

If Sam is depressed, give him some key messages about depression.

- Depression is common – many people (including people without prior mental health problems) experience feelings and difficulties just like those he has been experiencing.
- When people are depressed, they often stop doing things they enjoy. They also put off doing things they need to get done.
- Stopping fun things and putting off tasks makes people feel even worse, but starting to do them again can make them feel better. Show Sam Figure 8.1.
- Sam can actively help with recovering his usual mood, by becoming more active again.

Reviewing current activities and showing links with mood

Using the form in Table 8.1, help the person recall their activities on the previous day. Try to do it hour by hour, except for periods of extended activity of the same kind, such as sleep, which can be logged in a block. Ask if that day was different from the rest of the week and pay particular attention to the previous weekend. Note down activities that only occur on some days, and get the client to rate them using the same procedure as below.

The monitoring form has four columns. The first records the hour (or hours), the second the activity (or activities) and the third and fourth columns ask Sam to rate the activities for enjoyment and importance. Ratings for enjoyment and importance use an 11-point scale from 0 (not at all) to 10 (extremely). Activities can be enjoyable but not important or vice versa. Some activities will have similar ratings for enjoyment and importance. Use the form to show that the person's worst mood was when they were not enjoying themselves, and their better mood was when they achieved something or were doing something enjoyable.

Table 8.1   My activities.

Time	Activities on _____ day	Enjoyment 0 (not at all) −10 (extremely)	Importance 0 (not at all) −10 (extremely)

Place a tick (check mark) next to the time when your mood was best.
Place a cross next to the time when your mood was worst.
How does that relate to your activities?

When	Activities on other days	Enjoyment 0 (not at all) −10 (extremely)	Importance 0 (not at all) −10 (extremely)

Table 8.2 sets out Sam's initial rating with his practitioner as he did his best to reconstruct the previous day. Sam rated his sleep as not very enjoyable, because he was restless during the night and had some bad dreams. He rated it as reasonably important, because it is necessary but not helping him achieve anything. He rated the 30 minutes he spent showering and dressing as reasonably enjoyable. He quite likes standing in the shower but finding clothes and getting dressed are boring. He thought that, like sleep, it is just one of those things you have to do so it got a rating of 5 for importance. He spent an hour having breakfast and watching morning TV. He enjoyed his breakfast, which Angela made for him. He usually really enjoys food. Lately he has lost a bit of interest but it was still better than most things he did during the day. He always watches morning TV but does not pay much attention to what is on unless something really interesting has happened. He can't remember what was on yesterday morning. He rated breakfast the same as sleep and showering but because it was combined with TV, which was not important at all, he gave an overall rating of 3.

After breakfast, Angela asked him to take her dog for a walk and pick up some milk and cigarettes while she cleaned up. The dog really likes a walk. When Sam is feeling good, he takes the dog for quite a long walk. At present, he feels he barely has the energy to get to the shop. He knows it is good for his health to walk so he rated the activity as a bit more important than the things he had done so far that day. However, he could not say he enjoyed it. He does not like going into the shop. The old man who runs it looks at him strangely. The only thing he enjoys is watching Angela's dog sniffing about but even that irritates him at times. When he got home, he felt exhausted, even through the shop is only a few blocks away.

Table 8.2 Sam's first activity record.

Time	Activity	Enjoyment	Importance
12.00–8.30	Sleep	3	5
8.30–9.00	Shower and get dressed	5	5
9.00–10.00	Breakfast and TV	7	3
10.00–11.00	Walk the dog, buy milk and cigarettes	4	6
11.00–12.00 X	Lie down and call from mother	3	3
12.00–1.00	Can't remember – might have had a cup of coffee	7	2
1.00–2.00	Lunch – help Angela with the dishes	6	5
2.00–3.30 √	Replace tail light on Angela's car	7	8
3.30–5.00	Appointment with doctor and shopping with Angela	4	7
5.00–7.00	Can't remember – lie down	3	3
7.00–8.00	Prepare and eat dinner	6	5
8.00–8.30	Clean up after dinner	4	5
8.30–10.30	Watch DVD	5	3
10.30–12.30	Watch motor races on TV	8	2

Sam doesn't remember what happened when he got home, except that he had a lie-down for a while until the phone rang. It was his mother reminding him he had an appointment to see the doctor that afternoon. He talked briefly with her. She asked him how Angela was so he handed the phone over to Angela so she could tell her. They talked for a while and he lay down again. He does not like lying down during the day. It is very boring. He would not do it but he feels tired and can't think of anything else to do. He rated this period as 3 for both enjoyment and importance. Sam was quite hazy about the next hour. He rated it 2 for importance: 'can't have been important or I would remember something'. He thinks he probably had a coffee during this period: 'Angela always likes coffee in the middle of the day and asks me to make her one'. He quite enjoys drinking coffee and 'I don't mind making her one, because she does a lot for me'.

He thinks they had lunch between 1pm and 2pm. He remembers they had baked beans on toast because the beans stuck to the bottom of the saucepan when he was heating them. Angela asked him to stir them while she was making the toast but he forgot. She made a fuss about it but they weren't badly burned and tasted fine. After lunch, Angela washed the dishes and he dried them. They soaked the saucepan so it would be easier to wash at dinner time. He rated this period as a 6 for enjoyment. The beans were nice but drying dishes is pretty boring. Lunch is another of those things you have to do so it rated 5 for importance.

After lunch he replaced the tail light on Angela's car. The left-side brake light has not been working for a while and she was pulled over by the police the other day and told to fix it or the car would be certified unroadworthy. It took a while. The car is old and some of the screws were rusty. It was just a bulb that needed replacing but it took a while to find the right size. He likes working on cars. Even though it was an easy job, working out the best way to go about it, locating the right tools and sourcing the replacement part kept his mind occupied and for a while he forgot how he was feeling. He rated it as a 7 for enjoyment, 'it was the highlight of my day really', and 8 for importance, because having a defective brake light affects the safety of the vehicle and Angela has enough difficulty paying for fuel without having the cost of getting it recertified for roadworthiness.

Sam and Angela went out after fixing the car. While he saw the doctor, she went shopping. He had to wait half an hour to see the doctor and then it was in and out in 5–10 minutes. The doctor just asked a few questions about his depression and checked on whether he was experiencing side-effects from the medication. The doctor agreed that Sam was not show-ing much improvement but suggested they maintain the same medication and dose for another 3 weeks. He then met up with Angela and trailed around with her while she looked at clothes. He suggested to Angela that they have a coffee but she was concerned about money and said they could have coffee when they got home. All in all, the outing was very boring and he rated it as 4 for enjoyment. The only part of it he enjoyed was browsing through some car magazines in the doctor's waiting room. He rated the importance of the appointment at 7 because 'I guess they are trying to do something about my depression'.

Sam could not remember what happened in the next 2 hours. After he got home, he thinks he must have gone into the bedroom and laid down for a while. He does not recollect whether they had coffee when they got back but they might have. He rated this period the same as his morning lie-down. He remembers Angela coming into the bedroom around 7pm and asking him to help her cut up some vegetables. They had a bit of an argument when he suggested ordering in a pizza instead. Angela made soup with the vegetables and some lentils. It tasted good and was probably healthier than pizza. Cutting up vegetables was boring but easy enough. He rated the preparation and eating of dinner as 6 for enjoyment and 5 for importance. After dinner they cleaned up. Angela made him scrub the saucepan with the burnt beans that had been soaking all afternoon. That was easy enough. He rated the enjoyment of cleaning up as 4 and the importance as 5.

The rest of the night was spent watching television. Angela had rented a movie while they were out. It was OK but a 'chick-flic'. It was nice sitting on the couch with Angela with her snuggling up next to him. He rated the enjoyment as 7 and the importance as 6. It was nice doing something together and not arguing. He knows it was important to do some things she liked even if he was not very interested. After the DVD, Angela said she was feeling tired and went to bed. Sam decided to stay up and watch the motor races, which were on one of the cable channels. He likes motor races: 'you never know what will happen'. It was even more enjoyable than fixing Angela's car but not at all important: 'just killing time really'.

Sam went to bed around 12.30 but took a while to get to sleep. He does not remember how long. He woke up during the night and made himself a cup of tea but does not remember when or how long he was awake for.

When Sam thought about the time he felt worse, it was when he was lying down in the morning and was thinking about how boring his life was. He felt best when he fixed the tail light. The rehabilitation practitioner showed him Figure 8.1 again, and showed how his experience fitted the picture. Maybe if he could do more things that made him feel good, his depression might lift. Sam agreed but said it would be hard to get moving. His practitioner said they could go slowly to help him get moving. First, it may be a good idea to get a better picture of how things are now, so they could see when things get better. Also, they needed to look at what he'd like to do.

Some clients like Sam will be able to monitor their activities between sessions; if so, talk about why it will be important to keep track of what they have been doing, so they can see how it changes. Negotiate a time to fill in the daily monitoring record, e.g. 10 minutes at the end of the day might work. Get the client to set up some reminders – phones are perfect for this. Some clients prefer paper copies and others will work better with an electronic form. You might even be able to set up a personalised online form.

However, many if not most people with schizophrenia find this task difficult to remember, or find it hard to motivate themselves to do it. In those cases, use the next session to do another review of the previous day or two, or phone them during the next week to do a brief review of the previous day.

Review of activities

The next session should take place as soon as possible, but no later than a week after the previous session. If feasible, a follow-up session 3 days after the previous one is preferable.

If the client has been self-monitoring and comes with forms that are more or less fully completed, you have a great start to BA. However, don't be surprised if there are missing and/or incomplete forms. Depression affects both memory and motivation. When the depression is coupled with a condition such as schizophrenia, the obstacles are even greater. Try reconstructing the previous day, and ideally a day on the previous weekend, and look for days when the person undertook other activities. If you and Sam decide to keep trying self-monitoring, consider enlisting the support of a partner or family member, using different kinds of reminders or making small changes to the forms. Check motivation and use motivational strategies if the client is ambivalent. Be empathic but clear: 'I know these forms can be boring but it's essential that we discover some ways to help you feel better'.

If the client has not been self-monitoring, see if they can remember what they did the previous day, and (if possible) a day on the previous weekend. Ask if there were any days when they did other things; write those down or fill out a third form.

Review the patterns. How similar are the days? Are there certain times when more enjoyable or more important activities are likely to occur? When are the flat periods when nothing that is either enjoyable or important takes place? Review the best and worst mood on the previous day, and again relate moods to enjoyment and achievement.

Explore opportunities to increase the amount of enjoyable activity, the amount of important activity and the enjoyment of important activity. Use a brief checklist of activities like those in Figure 8.1 to identify ones the client would like to do more often (or start doing again). Use your knowledge of the client to help them add any other activities that are relevant to them.

If the client does not identify any tasks they want to get done, leave that for the moment and focus on things they may enjoy (Box 8.1). If they say they would not enjoy any activities, get them to identify ones they used to enjoy. Tell them that when they feel down, things may not be as much fun as usual but they may still help to lift their mood.

Box 8.1 Activities I'd like to do

Tick all the things you like doing – add others if you want. Circle any you'd like to do more often. Focus on the ones you like best. Then, tick any things that make you feel good when you get them done. Circle any you'd like to work on. Focus on ones you think you can do.

Things I like doing	Tasks that make me feel good when I get them done
☐ Phoning/texting a friend	☐ Getting up early
☐ Meeting up with a friend	☐ Making my bed
☐ Going to a café	☐ Cooking a meal
☐ Cooking	☐ Washing up
☐ Making music	☐ Cleaning up
☐ Doing exercise	☐ Getting groceries
☐ Going for a walk	☐ Going to work
☐ Riding a bike	☐ Keeping an appointment
☐ Swimming/surfing	☐ Paying bills
☐ Fun shopping	☐ Repairing/fixing something
☐ Playing with pets	☐ _____
☐ Playing sport	☐ _____
☐ Watching sports	☐ _____
☐ Reading	
☐ Listening to music	
☐ Watching TV	
☐ Having a bath	
☐ _____	
☐ _____	
☐ _____	

When Sam and his rehabilitation practitioner reviewed his daily monitoring forms, it was clear that he spent a lot of time in bed or lying down, and that he found this activity to be neither enjoyable nor important. It was also likely that the amount of time he spent lying down was making his sleep less enjoyable, because he typically woke for several hours during the night. He was in a vicious cycle. He rested during the day because he did not sleep well at night, but the amount of rest he had during the day meant that he was likely to be awake and alert for periods during the night. Finding things he could do instead of lying down was clearly a priority.

He said he wanted to start playing his guitar again, and would like to go to the football. He liked to go for coffee, and to have take-away meals. He also had some favourite CDs and TV shows.

Making a plan

If the client is committed to giving behavioural activation a try, it is important they understand the following.

- It will require some effort on their part – sometimes they won't feel like doing things they are asked to do.

Box 8.2   My plan

What I'll do
When I'll do it
What I need to do to beforehand
How I'll remember to do it

- It may take a little time before they notice that they are feeling better.
- Fun activities may not be as much fun as normal, and things they achieve may not feel as good, because they are feeling low. The important thing is not to focus on whether they feel as good as they usually would, but on the fact that they feel much better than if they didn't do them.
- There will probably be some set-backs – they may feel they are getting better but then slip back to feeling bad again, before they achieve a more stable recovery.
- You may make some mistakes – sometimes pushing them too hard, sometimes not hard enough. If they don't do an activity, it is not a failure on their part – you got it wrong. This message may help to prevent them feeling bad or giving up when things don't quite go to plan.
- It might be helpful if someone else is involved – at least some of the time; if they know what the client is working on, they can support and encourage them.

If the client is reluctant, try and find out what is holding them back. They may feel the therapy won't make any difference. If this is the case, point to the experience reported by Mairs *et al.* (2011): 'As the weeks went by I found myself, you know, doing a bit more. And I'd a sense of achievement, you know, accomplishment, I'd done something and I'd feel, you know, I'd feel it was worthwhile, and that, keep meself (*sic*) healthy' (p.498).

The client may feel they don't have the energy to do anything. If this is the case, emphasise that you will only expect them to do small things while they are feeling that way. The important thing when recovering from depression is not to do major things but to start taking some positive steps. If they are worried about failure, they may also be concerned about disappointing you, or other people. If this is the case, tell them that, whatever the outcome, no-one will be disappointed if they have done their best.

Use the form in Box 8.2 to plan to do 1–2 activities today and tomorrow; usually, it is best to focus initially on ones lasting 5–30 minutes. Help the client fill out the plan for each activity they are going to try.

Behavioural activation uses standard behavioural principles of shaping behaviour through positive reinforcement of small changes. In most cases, this involves noticing an increase in activity, and the pleasure that comes from doing fun things and completing tasks. You, and other people like Sam's girlfriend, can help Sam notice his achievements, and how much better he feels when he does things he likes. The focus is on small changes, so that the person feels good about what he has achieved.

To reduce inactivity, some concrete rewards may sometimes be needed but try to negotiate them to be just a strategy to get started. If the alternative activity is to continue over a longer period, it needs to be sustained by natural or 'intrinsic' rewards (being fun to do, giving satisfaction, receiving thanks from others, etc.). It is important that we don't reward an activity that is intrinsically pleasurable otherwise Sam may think he only did it because of another reward.

Sam was averaging 2 hours of lying down each day (not counting overnight). He thought he could reduce this to 90 minutes per day without too much difficulty. He wanted to use the time to get some housework done, but he didn't think the satisfaction of finishing that would be rewarding enough for him to give up the 30 minutes of rest.

Rewards can be difficult to decide on. A reward has to be valuable enough to make it seem worthwhile to undertake the activity (e.g. giving up 30 minutes lying down each day), but something that can be delivered in small doses.

Sam and his rehabilitation practitioner (with Angela's support) agreed that the reward would be order-in pizza after 6 days with 90 minutes or less lie-down time during the day. The days did not have to be successive, to allow for the possibility that he would have one or more 'bad' days. The rehabilitation practitioner worked with Sam to design and print some 'pizza certificates' that Angela would sign. Other possible rewards for Sam included going to a local football match. Sam and Angela will consider whether to do that instead in the second week. Note that the pizza, the football match and receiving the 'certificates' are also pleasurable events that will help to lift Sam's mood.

Review how the plan went

Within the next 3 days, contact the client (e.g. by phone) and see how the initial activities went. If they did the activities, ask how enjoyable and how important they were (using the 0–10 ratings). Help them to identify what they want to do between now and the next session. Ask them to write it down if they can, as you talk it through.

If they did not do the activities, find out what went wrong. Was the activity insufficiently enjoyable or important? If so, see if another activity might be better. Is an external reward needed? Try to find one. Was more preparation needed? Try to solve any challenges together. If this is difficult over the phone, reassure the client that there are often some difficulties in getting started, and say you can work on them together when you next meet up. Make an appointment within the next few days if possible.

Life areas, values and activities

In the next session, review daily activities over the previous week. Note changes to activity patterns, especially to activities that were targeted for change. Praise achievements and explore reasons for any non-achievement. Address barriers and remind the client that changing established patterns of behaviour is rarely straightforward and setbacks or difficulties are to be expected. If there was no movement at all in the direction of the change, the target may be too ambitious and it might be sensible to scale back or target a different activity for change. Note changes to ratings of enjoyment or importance of daily activity.

Activities will be most successfully sustained if they are consistent with the person's values and goals. Once the client is regularly doing some new activities, spend a session

Table 8.3 My values and goals.

Life area	Values/goals	Activities
Relationships: family, friends and/or partner		
Education/career: both current and future. Includes voluntary work, caring responsibilities		
Recreation/interests: this life area refers to leisure time, whether active (e.g. sports, hobbies) or passive (reading, movies) and whether alone or with others		
Mind/body/spirituality: physical and mental health as well as religion and/or spirituality		
Daily responsibilities: self-care, household maintenance		

mapping their values and goals and identifying some activities that will be steps towards goals. A simple form (Table 8.3) is used to structure this process and to maintain an ongoing record.

This form is a working document that will be developed and modified in later sessions. Activities will be added and deleted in the light of experience. An electronic version will make it easy to modify. For many clients, it will be best to start with 1–2 domains. Attempting to complete the form in one sitting may otherwise be overwhelming for clients who have given a lot of thought to their values or goals, let alone activities that relate to them.

Sam's rehabilitation practitioner introduced the life areas, values and activities form by saying: 'The purpose of this form is to get a better understanding of what is important to you and what you would like to achieve in different areas of your life. Some you might already be clear about and others you might not have thought about much. Let's start with one or two areas of your life where you already have some ideas about what you would like to achieve'.

She then gave Sam a copy of the form and explained how it was set out, with five life areas and spaces for setting out values and goals and current and future activities for each life area.

Sam was able to identify some values and/or goals in each of the areas but had more difficulty with activities that might be linked to these goals. The only activities from his recent records that he could see were clearly linked with values or goals were making coffee for Angela, going shopping with Angela, repairing the tail light on Angela's car and helping Angela prepare dinner. With a little prompting, he could also see that attending his doctor's appointments and working on his BA programme was good for his mental health.

Values and goals provide the basis for planning future activities. It is important, where possible, to anchor any goals in core values. Values are both stable and important. Goals that are closely linked to core values are likely to persist and the associated activities are likely to be maintained even when they require effort. Sometimes people have difficulty articulating values. When Sam was asked what was important to him about his family, he came up with 'I wish mum didn't worry so much about me'. This is neither a value nor a goal but implies both (e.g. making mum happier), and it has sufficient links to both to generate meaningful and important activities. When Sam was asked what might help his mum feel less worried, he said: 'She always worries when I don't call her or drop by. She phones up and talks to Angela. Angela is good at talking with her on the phone. I never know what to say. It is better if I drop by. She makes me a cup of tea and we talk about a few things. I haven't felt like it lately, but I guess it is something I could do – and I know it would make her feel less worried'.

Sam and his rehabilitation worker noted this in the activities column. Dates and times were specifically noted to help with monitoring.

There were some life areas where Sam could not think of any activities, even though he had some values or goals. It is not essential to have all life areas with planned activities by the end of this session. The record is maintained and developed over time. The role of the practitioner is to make sure the client is mindful of each life area. A good message is: 'It is good to have planned activities across a range of life areas – not all your plans will work out so having plans for several different areas makes it more likely you will have success in one or more'.

When the client identifies a complex activity, it is important to break it down into a series of specific smaller activities. If they generate a lot of activities, rank them for difficulty. As a general rule, it is best to start with ones that are relatively simple.

The session should end with at least one agreed planned activity to be implemented in the next week. Sam undertook to visit his mum. This was a simple (but not necessarily easy) activity. All that was required was to schedule a date and time. He also wanted to do something about the sound system in Angela's car. It sounded awful and even she complained about it. This was a much more complex activity that involved negotiating with Angela the type of sound system she wanted, locating specific examples, purchasing and installing. Sam decided he needed to have a discussion with Angela about the kind of sound system she would like to have in her car. This would include some research on eBay to get an idea of costs and maybe a visit to a retailer so she could get a better idea about the look, sound and features. Sam was confident he could get a better deal online and maybe pick up a good second-hand system but after some discussion with his rehabilitation practitioner, he agreed that Angela would not be happy if she did not have a good understanding of what he was planning to get for her (especially as she would be paying for it).

Check for anticipated enjoyment of the activities. If anticipated enjoyment is low, introducing a reward may be worthwhile. In this case, Sam thought researching car sound systems would have an enjoyment rating of 6–7 but visiting his mum was more likely 4 because he rarely feels like going out these days. His rehabilitation practitioner discussed rewards but Sam decided he would do it because it was the right thing to do, even if he did not feel like it.

It may help to have a specific form with scheduled activities.

Integrate the activity record with life areas, values and activities

By the next session, the activity record should contain a mix of previous activities, ones derived from the initial review of fun activities and tasks, and ones from the life areas, values and activities form. Some key issues include the following.

- To what extent were the new activities implemented?
- What, if any, barriers were experienced when trying new activities?
- How were the new activities rated for enjoyment?
- How were the new activities rated for importance?
- Which existing activities were sacrificed to make way for the new activities?

When activities are successfully implemented, check for intrinsic reward. Intrinsic reward will be greatest when activities are rated high for both enjoyment and importance. The practitioner can show the client that they are impressed by achievement with statements such as: 'you really managed that well' or 'that was a pretty tough assignment but you handled it well'. When activities are not successfully implemented, it is possible that the difficulty was greater than anticipated and a simpler activity should be tried first. The practitioner should accept responsibility for failure in such circumstances with statements such as: 'I think I underestimated how difficult that would be' or 'I didn't take into account … when I suggested you try …'. However, as discussed above, the activity may not have had sufficient intrinsic reward, and some kind of extrinsic reward might be necessary to overcome initial resistance to undertaking the activity.

Discuss and identify new activities that are consistent with values and goals. Where possible, scheduled activities should be spread across different life areas.

Subsequent sessions

Subsequent sessions build on the groundwork done in the initial sessions. The aim is to increase the amount of activity and, in particular, increase activity that is pleasurable or important or both. BA should not be a drudge and it is important to schedule some activities likely to be enjoyable even though not important.

Expect variable rates of progress and fluctuating motivation. BA requires patience and persistence in the practitioner. Consider charting mean enjoyment and importance scores from daily monitoring records (see Figure 8.2).

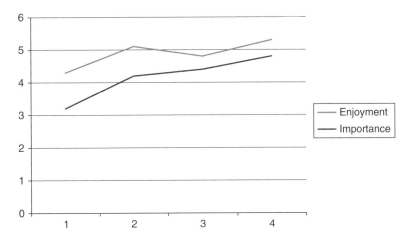

Figure 8.2 A chart of client progress.

Self-monitoring is difficult to maintain for long periods. The emphasis of the rehabilitation is on changes in activities rather than on filling in forms. Focus on achievement of behavioural goals, and sample daily changes in activity at regular intervals (e.g. monthly) using a week of self-monitoring or sampled days reconstructed within sessions. Help the client identify new behaviours to try, and (if they are progressing well) develop further steps towards their goals, so they do not become bored and continue to have a sense of achievement. However, keep track of their symptomatic status; if they are finding BA stressful or are going through a period of increased risk of relapse, help them focus on less challenging (but still enjoyable) activities.

Ending a behavioural activation programme

Behavioural activation is time limited. Mairs *et al.* (2011) allowed a period of 6 months for a pilot with people affected by severe mental illness and found that participants attended an average of 14 sessions during that period. We suggest that practitioners provide some further education about depression when ending formal BA sessions. In particular, it is important to point out that depression is often recurrent and that it is helpful to detect it early and counter it with strategies learned during the BA programme, especially behaviour monitoring and activity scheduling. It is also worth encouraging the client to contact you for a booster session from time to time. If a client is receiving case management from another practitioner, it is worth providing the case manager with some information about BA so that the case manager can encourage re-engagement if and when the need arises.

Supplementing behavioural activation with cognitive interventions

A cognitive approach to BA uses it to address negative thoughts that are also feeding into depression. These thoughts also make it harder for the person to start BA, and in some cases have already been mentioned above, e.g. 'Changing my activities won't do any good'; 'I am a complete failure, I'll never succeed at anything, there is no point in trying'. Up to now, we have addressed them only via problem solving potential difficulties or considering others' experiences.

In cognitive therapy, the BA activities are used as a behavioural experiment, to test out overly negative thoughts. This is a much more powerful approach to them. Ask the client what might happen if the thought is true. Try to set up the experiment so it is hard for it not to succeed. Then, as soon as possible after the person makes an attempt, when you are looking at their progress, remind them about their prediction and note that it did not come true. They will probably try to find a way to rescue their thought (e.g. 'I wouldn't have succeeded without the help of my girlfriend' or 'I only succeeded because the task was really easy'). Acknowledge that, but help them find a more realistic thought (e.g. 'I can succeed some of the time, if I have some help, or the task isn't too hard'). Progressive experiments like this, where the person attempts harder tasks, can eliminate some of the provisos and help establish a more positive thought pattern. Get them to rehearse this thought whenever they notice the negative one (e.g. 'I can succeed at things most of the time, as long as I do them step by step'); ask them to try to recall their recent attempts and how successful (or pleasurable) they were. This will not only help to ensure that they keep trying, it will also help to lift their mood further.

Another cognitive intervention involves teaching mindfulness – in this case, a simple version, where the person notices their sensations and emotions. Show them how to track what they are seeing, hearing, touching and feeling in their body, and what emotions or pleasure that makes them experience. Then get them to try doing this when they are undertaking a pleasurable activity or have a sense of achievement. This will increase the positive effects of the activity, and will also tend to distract them from negative thoughts that may undercut the impact of the activity.

Tips for behavioural activation

- Patience and perseverance are the keys to BA – don't expect rapid progress in the beginning.
- Small steps and small successes are important.
- Some daily monitoring is essential, but can be done in sessions.
- Where appropriate, enlist the support of partners, family members and friends.
- Break down complex activities into manageable, achievable tasks.
- Maintain the focus on activities that are enjoyable and/or important.
- Progress is rarely linear – prepare yourself and your client for setbacks.
- Refer regularly to values and goals – and use values and goals to assist with motivation.
- Use extraneous rewards when intrinsic rewards are inadequate.

References

Buckley PF, Miller BJ, Lehrer DS, Castle DJ (2009) *Psychiatric comorbidities and schizophrenia. Schizophrenia Bulletin* **35**, 383.

Cuijpers P, van Straten A, Warmerdam L (2007) Behavioral activation treatments for depression: a meta-analysis. *Clinical Psychology Review* **27**, 318–26.

Dimidjian S, Barrera M Jr, Martell C, Muñoz RF, Lewinsohn PM (2011) The origins and current status of behavioral activation treatments for depression. *Annual Review of Clinical Psychology* **7**, 1–38.

Furtado VA, Srihari V (2008) Atypical antipsychotics for people with both schizophrenia and depression. *Cochrane Database of Systematic Reviews* **1**, CD005377

Lejuez CW, Hopko DR, Acierno R, Daughters SB, Pagoto SL (2011) Ten year revision of the brief behavioral activation treatment for depression: revised treatment manual. *Behavior Modification* **35**, 111–61.

Mairs H, Lovell K, Campbell M, Keeley P (2011) Development and pilot investigation of behavioral activation for negative symptoms. *Behavior Modification* **35**, 486–506.

Sturmey P (2009) Behavioral activation is an evidence-based treatment for depression. *Behavior Modification* **33**, 818–29.

Whitehead C, Moss S, Cardno A, Lewis G (2003) Antidepressants for the treatment of depression in people with schizophrenia: a systematic review. *Psychological Medicine* **33**, 589–99.

Chapter 9

Cognitive Remediation

Hamish J. McLeod and Robert King

> Sam has been complaining a lot about his concentration and memory of late: 'I forget appointments and sometimes I can't remember whether or not I have taken my medication. If I am watching a movie on TV I keep losing the story line and I have to get my girlfriend to explain what has happened – which really annoys me, and her. It has been bad ever since I started taking medication but it seems to be getting worse. It worries me because I would really like to get a job and earn some money – or at least do some training – and I don't see how I could manage any kind of job the way I am at the moment.'

As Sam's case manager or rehabilitation worker, how can you help him?

Step 1: start with some psychoeducation

Episodes of mental illness can lead to significant changes in social and occupational roles. These very real losses can erode self-esteem and diminish expectations of a positive future. In addition, stigma and shame may further demoralise the person and undermine active efforts to change. Psychoeducation that normalises the person's lived experience but also instils hope is a critical first step in promoting engagement in active rehabilitation.

There are four important messages for Sam.

- Problems with concentration and memory are very common among people affected by mental illness – you are not on your own with this and these problems do not mean that a person is weak or lazy.
- Pessimistic thoughts and feeling demoralised about the prospect of recovery can undermine attempts to change and this might lead to giving up. Getting structured help and support from another person is sometimes a necessary first step to help take back control of one's life.
- The problems may not be anything to do with the medication – you started the medication around the time it became clear you were developing a mental illness so the problems are just as likely to be caused by the illness itself as the medication.

Manual of Psychosocial Rehabilitation, First Edition. Edited by Robert King, Chris Lloyd, Tom Meehan, Frank P. Deane and David J. Kavanagh.
© 2012 Blackwell Publishing Ltd. Published 2012 by Blackwell Publishing Ltd.

- Regardless of whether the problems are caused by the illness, the medications or both, you can work on your memory and concentration, develop your capacity with both and greatly improve your chances of success with work and study.

Step 2: get an accurate baseline assessment

You and Sam both need to know the nature and extent of his concentration and memory problems. It is also sensible to identify his other cognitive strengths and weaknesses as well as his level of insight into his cognitive difficulties. Determining the level of insight becomes very important when the person underestimates or overestimates their level of impairment. Underestimation may feed demoralisation because of a tendency to set unreasonably ambitious goals and overestimation of deficits can decrease motivation and promote apathy. Many useful assessment tools are now available in the public domain and can be used by any appropriately qualified mental health worker. The use of others may be restricted to specially qualified practitioners.

Neuropsychological assessment

One way of determining Sam's relative cognitive strengths and weaknesses is to get a full neuropsychological assessment. This is a very thorough assessment, using sophisticated standardised measures, that provides a detailed profile of cognitive functioning. It is the best means of evaluating cognitive deficits but it is not always feasible as it depends on the availability of appropriate specialists and may be costly.

If you do not have access to someone who can conduct a neuropsychological assessment, we recommend the use of some of the measures discussed in Chapter 2 of this book (e.g. the Brief Assessment of Cognition in Schizophrenia; BACS). There are two excellent resources by Lezak et al. (2004) and Strauss et al. (2006) that contain comprehensive descriptions of a large variety of cognitive tests, organised according to the cognitive domain under evaluation. Some widely used tests such as the Rey Auditory Verbal Learning Test and the Trail Making Test are in the public domain and the materials, instructions and norms can be obtained directly from the books. Others such as the Symbol Digit Modalities Test are quite inexpensive. These tests do not require extensive training for effective use but we recommend completing a number of practice trials with friends and colleagues to ensure scores are not affected by clumsiness in administration of the test. When possible, use tests that have parallel or multiple equivalent forms. This reduces the chance that any improvements seen with repeat assessments over time are attributable to practice effects.

A complementary approach that is a less resource-intensive alternative to formal neuropsychological testing is to use an interview-based measure of cognitive functioning. Measures such as the Clinical Global Impression of Cognition in Schizophrenia (CGI-CogS; Ventura et al., 2008) and the Schizophrenia Cognition Rating Scale (SCoRS, available from the author on request – richard.keefe@duke.edu) (Keefe et al., 2006) have been developed specifically to assess the types of subjective cognitive complaints that affect daily functioning in people with schizophrenia. An important feature of these measures is that they require the practitioner to obtain input from someone who knows the person with schizophrenia well enough to comment on their levels of cognitive difficulty. This can reveal discrepancies between the person's subjective abilities and their actual level of functioning. Even if a formal interview measure is not used, it is good practice to gain collateral information from a third party. This should be done at the initial assessment and repeated at regular intervals during the remediation programme.

If it is difficult to access either a neuropsychologist or a standardised test you can administer yourself, we recommend you encourage Sam to use a website such as http://cognitivefun.net/. This site contains a neat set of online tests and allows the user to maintain a record of performance. (Most of these sites require the user to create an account and log on each time in order for progress data to accumulate. If you are going to use this method of monitoring improvements over time, it is important that you ensure that the patient understands that they need to log in each time they complete a training session.) There are also some similar tests on http://cognitivelabs.com, although this is a more commercial site and does not allow the same easy monitoring of performance. Other websites that offer online recording of performance are provided at the end of this chapter.

Assessment of awareness of cognitive deficits

It is well known that people with schizophrenia can display different levels of insight into their symptoms such as delusions and hallucinations. However, they can also show varying awareness of their cognitive abilities (Medalia & Lim, 2004) and difficulties with day-to-day functioning (Bowie *et al.*, 2007). Substantial discrepancies between subjective ratings of difficulties, those provided by mental health workers and the results of structured tests are common. These discrepancies may impinge on the person's motivation to engage in a remediation programme and so it is advisable to assess their level of awareness before commencing treatment.

A number of scales have been developed to assess the subjective awareness of cognitive deficits in people with schizophrenia. For example, the Subjective Scale to Investigate Cognition in Schizophrenia (SSTICS; Stip *et al.*, 2003) is a 21-item self-report questionnaire that addresses impairments of memory, attention, executive function, language and motor abilities. The items address cognitive problems that will impair everyday functioning (e.g. 'Do you forget to take your medication?' and 'Do you have difficulty memorising things such as a grocery list or a list of names?') rated on a five-point Likert scale (from 'never' to 'very often'), with higher scores indicating more frequent problems. This type of measure will be particularly useful with people like Sam who can recognise that they have some cognitive problems.

However, when there is less agreement about the presence, nature and extent of any cognitive difficulties, it will be appropriate to use a measure that incorporates the practitioner's judgement about the person's level of awareness of their difficulties. The Measure of Insight into Cognition – Clinician Rated (MIC-CR; the MIC-CR record form and manual are available on request from Dr Alice Medalia – am2938@columbia.edu) (Medalia & Thysen, 2008) is a 12-item semi-structured interview specifically designed to index insight into cognitive deficits in people with schizophrenia. The structure and response format are similar to those used in the Scale for the Assessment of Unawareness of Mental Disorder (SUMD; Amador *et al.*, 1993) and the items assess both the recognition of a problem (e.g. awareness of trouble listening or paying attention) and the beliefs about the cause of the problem (e.g. it is due to mental illness, it is possibly related to mental illness, or it is unrelated to mental illness). In Sam's case, his assertion that the problems with concentration and memory started when he was first prescribed medication indicates some ambivalence about attributing his cognitive symptoms to the effects of schizophrenia.

Assessment of the functional impact of cognitive deficits

One of the main challenges with cognitive remediation programmes is getting the effects to generalise beyond the exercises and drills to 'real-world' outcomes such as the capacity for effective work or studying (Wykes & Huddy, 2009). There is some evidence that generalised benefits will be enhanced when cognitive remediation is provided in conjunction with interventions that target the achievement of meaningful life goals such as vocational rehabilitation (Bell *et al.*, 2008). Hence, an important part of the assessment process will be identifying behavioural outcomes that will be meaningful in the everyday life of the person with schizophrenia. This may be done informally by discussing the goals that the person wants to achieve when they have completed the remediation program or via the use of structured assessments that identify areas of functional strength and weakness.

One simple strategy for determining the general impact of cognitive deficits on daily functioning is to scrutinise the responses to items on the CGI-CogS and SCoRS described above. Other options that are freely available in the published literature include the five-item Patient Perception of Functioning Scale (Ehmann *et al.*, 2007) and the 14-item Life Functioning Questionnaire (Altshuler *et al.*, 2002). However, a number of scales have now been subject to expert review to determine their suitability for measuring 'real-world' functioning in people with schizophrenia (Leifker *et al.*, 2011). Leifker *et al.*'s study refined an initial pool of 59 measures down to four scales that are currently the most strongly endorsed by expert clinical practitioners and researchers. Two are hybrid measures that assess both everyday living skills and social functioning: the Heinrichs-Carpenter Quality of Life Scale (Heinrichs *et al.*, 1984) and the Specific Levels of Functioning Scale (SLOF; Schneider & Struening, 1983). The other two measures that received strong expert endorsement are primarily measures of social functioning: the Social Functioning Scale (Birchwood *et al.*, 1990) and the Social Behaviour Schedule (Wykes & Sturt, 1986). All of these measures can be administered by trained mental health professionals and provide comprehensive everyday functioning data that complement information about cognitive deficits obtained from formal neuropsychological testing.

The rehabilitation practitioner applied the BACS with Sam and found that his scores were substantially weaker than those of a normative population the same age in all areas. The pattern of results is presented in Table 9.1. He had moderate weaknesses in working memory, motor speed, verbal fluency, and reasoning and problem solving and more severe deficits in verbal memory and attention and processing speed.

Table 9.1 Sam's raw scores and standardised Z-scores on BACS subtests.

Subtest	Cognitive domain	Raw score	Deviation from normative average Z-scores						
			−3	−2	−1	0	+1	+2	+3
List Learning	Verbal Memory	28							
Digit Sequencing	Working Memory	17							
Token Motor Task	Motor Speed	65							
Verbal Fluency	Processing Speed	42							
Tower Test	Reasoning and Problem Solving	15							
Symbol Coding	Attention and Processing Speed	37							

Normative data taken from Keefe *et al.* (2008).

As Sam's case manager or rehabilitation worker, where do you go from here? Before introducing the cognitive remediation tasks, you need to address any attitudes, beliefs or gaps in understanding that might impair Sam's sustained engagement with the programme. This should be done in a collaborative way that conveys the possibility for improvement and models a systematic approach to problem solving. As a practitioner, you should remember that Sam will learn a lot of valuable skills from seeing how you help him break down his difficulties into manageable subtasks and goals. This will potentially occur in all the interactions you have with him, even if you are not explicitly working on any cognitive remediation exercises.

Step 3: some further psychoeducation

Start by sharing the findings with Sam. It is likely that he will be reassured that the tests confirm he really does have a problem and it is not his imagination or proof that he is just 'lazy'. However, he will also be worried that the problem may be irreversible, especially as he feels it is getting worse. For this reason you need to communicate some additional key messages.

- All of these cognitive functions can be improved.
- The brain, which controls all these functions, can respond to regular exercise and get fitter, like the rest of your body.
- Mental illness can weaken some areas of functioning, especially when the brain has been deprived of the stimulation it needs to keep fit and active.
- A brain 'workout' can be tiring and challenging but it can also be fun and interesting.
- It is important to develop the habit of doing some systematic brain exercise every day.

Step 4: check motivational level

Because cognitive remediation is demanding, Sam will need to have at least moderately strong motivation to improve his cognitive functioning. It is clear that he is already beyond the precontemplation stage in his readiness to change but is he ready for action or is he still just contemplating? If Sam seems a little ambivalent or uncertain, we suggest you apply some of the techniques set out in Chapter 6 until he is clearly ready for action. It is also very relevant for mental health workers to bear in mind the difference between intrinsic and extrinsically motivated behaviour. Extrinsic motivation refers to situations where behaviour is maintained primarily by the presence of external reinforcers such as monetary reward or social approval from others. These can be powerful sources of behavioural control in all walks of life but are vulnerable to the disappearance of the desired behaviour once the reinforcer is withdrawn. For example, consider how long you would continue in your current job if your employer suddenly stopped paying you. In contrast, intrinsic motivation refers to reinforcers of behaviour that are more 'internal' to the person such as enjoyment, satisfaction, sense of accomplishment, autonomy or competence. These types of reinforcer tap into a basic human preference for self-determination and help maintain behaviours over time even though access to externally provided reinforcers may change (Ryan & Deci, 2000; Vansteenkiste & Sheldon, 2006). This is critical in rehabilitation settings where the aim is to help the person establish new patterns of behaving that will be maintained even when the practitioner stops providing active treatment.

The recognition that enhancing intrinsic motivation is a critical goal of cognitive remediation programmes has highlighted the benefit of explicitly measuring motivation to engage in cognitive remediation (Choi *et al.*, 2010). Choi *et al.* have developed the Intrinsic Motivation Inventory, a 21-item self-report scale that captures the key concept of how much a person finds cognitive remediation tasks interesting and/or enjoyable (e.g. 'This activity was fun to do'; 'I would describe this activity as very interesting'). The

---

Why are we confident that cognitive remediation will help Sam?

The effectiveness of cognitive remediation for people with a diagnosis of mental illness has been researched by high-quality research teams in the US, UK and Europe. These studies have investigated a wide range of approaches to remediation from computerised programs to low-technology pen-and-paper activities and board games. The findings are consistent and robust: regular systematic cognitive exercises reliably enhance cognitive functioning. Even more importantly, there is established evidence that cognitive remediation, especially when integrated with a well-designed functional rehabilitation programme, enhances everyday functioning, including work capacity.

A meta-analysis by Wykes *et al.* (2011) identified 40 acceptable quality studies and found that cognitive remediation yielded:

> durable effects on global cognition and functioning ... No treatment element (remediation approach, duration, computer use, etc.) was associated with cognitive outcome. Cognitive remediation therapy was more effective when patients were clinically stable. Significantly stronger effects on functioning were found when cognitive remediation therapy was provided together with other psychiatric rehabilitation, and a much larger effect was present when a strategic approach was adopted together with adjunctive rehabilitation. (p.472)

Altogether, the research suggests that, while any regular purposeful challenging mental activity is likely to be helpful, a programme of specifically designed graduated cognitive exercises is likely to be even more helpful. Regular practice and understanding the connection between the exercises and daily life are also important components.

scale also indicates how much the person feels they are completing the tasks because they choose to and how valuable or useful they found the tasks. High scorers on this measure have been shown to attend more remediation sessions and engage with the tasks at a higher level of intensity. Using this measure may help identify beliefs and attitudes that indicate the need for more work using motivational interviewing strategies prior to starting a remediation programme.

Step 5: designing and beginning a brain workout programme

There are a number of different approaches to cognitive remediation in the published literature. The main points of variation are:

- the nature of the tasks (e.g. computer based versus paper and pencil)
- the degree of input from a practitioner
- the duration, frequency and intensity of the treatment sessions.

These issues are dealt with in more detail below but first, it is relevant to consider the conceptual aims of cognitive remediation. The practitioner can use this to guide the way in which they interact with the person receiving the treatment even if they are engaged in a variety of tasks and activities.

One of the fundamental reasons for the development of cognitive remediation is the recognition that people with schizophrenia experience significant cognitive difficulties and these impair community functioning more than the classic psychotic symptoms of delusions and hallucinations (Wykes & van der Gaag, 2001). Encouragingly, recent research into neuroplasticity has indicated that the brain can form new connections and regain some lost functions provided that the appropriate environmental stimulation is given. Cognitive remediation programmes are a structured way of providing the appropriate input at a level of intensity that increases the chance of enduring change. This stimulation can target very basic cognitive processes such as reaction time, sustained attention or processing speed or it can be focused on more complex cognitive abilities such as problem solving or accurately interpreting the emotional state and intentions of other people. A simple schematic model of these levels of cognition and their relationship to complex behaviour is presented in Figure 9.1.

Basic cognitive processes such as reacting quickly to stimuli and holding information in working memory are best trained through repetition and the computer-based tasks available on the internet are excellent for this type of drill-based training. Helping a person to improve their abilities in these domains provides the building blocks for improving higher level abilities. However, more complex tasks, such as solving novel problems and applying what has been learned across various situations, are harder to simulate on computer programs. These behaviourally and cognitively complex skills improve best with repeated practice in everyday life and so the rehabilitation worker should aim to start with achievable tasks that target basic cognitive processes and then gradually introduce more complex challenges that are based on real-world problems and challenges faced by the individual. For Sam, this might involve starting by helping him extend his

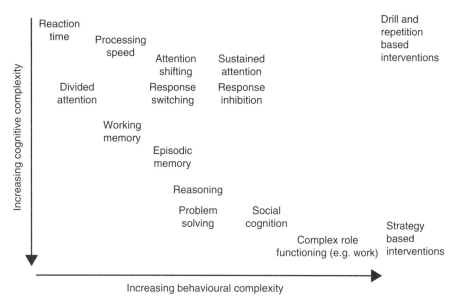

Figure 9.1   Schematic representation of different levels of cognition targeted in cognitive remediation.

concentration span and short-term memory and then moving on to more complex abilities such as strengthening his prospective memory so that he remembers to take his medication.

What are the best tasks to use?

One of the important findings from scientifically designed studies of cognitive remediation is that a wide variety of exercises and strategies show evidence of effectiveness and these effects are broadly equivalent across tasks (Wykes *et al.*, 2011). Furthermore, it is not clear that specific tasks affect specific cognitive domains (Grynszpan *et al.*, 2011). Rather, any kind of systematic cognitive training is likely to have positive impacts on several cognitive domains. This means you should not need a lot of sophisticated or complex equipment or software and it should be possible to negotiate with Sam the kind of workout that he can manage and is likely to enjoy. However, it is important that you help Sam to sustain his motivation and effectively transfer any improvements into his everyday life. The following principles are important.

- Start with simple tasks – early exercises should be easy to understand and easy to complete. If you are using an internet-based programme you should make sure that Sam understands how to log on to the site and navigate through the various test options. Make sure that you aim for errorless learning so that you pitch tasks at a level that will give Sam a very high chance of success. Simple motor reaction time tasks and working memory exercises (such as remembering strings of numbers) may be a good starting point. The exercises available at http://cognitivefun.net and playwithyourmind.com cover these basic abilities very well. Also, simple card games like Snap promote attention and motor speed.

- Keep practice sessions brief at the beginning: 15–20 minutes in total for each daily practice session for the first couple of weeks.
- Ensure there is variety but not too much complexity when starting out; each early session should contain 2–3 different tasks.
- Include at least one task that Sam reports as being fun to do.
- Build exercises around specific areas that matter to Sam, for example, a memory activity that will help him get better at keeping track of TV shows coming up that he wants to watch.
- Keep up the challenges. Once Sam has achieved mastery at one level, introduce a more complex or demanding task. Many of the online training programmes are designed to increase the difficulty of the tasks as the person improves.
- Widen the workout repertoire. When concentration and attention are better developed, move to higher order tasks such as memory development and planning.

You will find a list of resources that provide a wide variety of tasks at the end of this chapter.

Step 6: sustaining a brain workout programme

As case manager or rehabilitation worker, you should think of yourself as Sam's personal trainer. What this means in practice is that you need to motivate him, keep him on task and encourage him to sometimes go beyond his comfort zone. You also need to monitor his progress and make decisions about the focus of his brain workouts. Bear in mind that Sam will have setbacks, including times when he gets fed up with the whole process. Here are some tips that will help Sam keep at his programme.

- Feedback – monthly measurement will provide Sam with clear evidence that he is making gains. Remember that as with any kind of measurement, you have to make sure that the conditions at time of measurement are broadly equivalent. Do not conduct repeat assessments if Sam is acutely distressed as this will distort results.
- Link workout exercises to activities that are meaningful to Sam. If Sam wants to get a job or undertake a training course, discuss with him how the workout is building his capacity to achieve on work or study tasks. Sam had noticed that he was missing appointments and could not remember if he had taken his medication – check if this is still a problem. These real-world goals should be written down for Sam to refer to when he is feeling less motivated to persevere with the training programme.
- Help Sam identify everyday activities that will help him build his capacity. These might range from mentally adding up the costs of purchases before reaching the cash register to working on crossword or Sudoku puzzles in the daily newspaper.
- Rewards – while building capacity is inherently rewarding, it can be helpful to build in external rewards for undertaking more challenging tasks (see Chapter 8). Sam's family have an investment in his success and might like to get involved in scheduling some rewards. Remember, rewards do not need to be large to be effective.

Step 7: integrating cognitive remediation with a broader rehabilitation programme

Cognitive remediation is most effective when it is well integrated into a rehabilitation programme designed to assist the client to meet their recovery goals (Wykes *et al.*, 2011). This step does not have to wait until the end of the cognitive remediation programme. Integration should take place from the beginning as this helps maintain motivation when doing repetitive and sometimes boring exercises. It also helps the client to make use of and practise developing cognitive skills throughout the week.

Sam has indicated that he would like to work and this would be an excellent basis for integration focus in this case. However, cognitive functioning is central to a wide range of activities and integration can be achieved regardless of whether the client goals are to make friends, learn the guitar or even enjoy television. The key features of integration are as follows.

- Identify some of the important cognitive challenges associated with the client's goals. For example, even simple jobs require attention and concentration and capacity to remember instructions.
- Identify routine daily activities that involve similar challenges. These can provide a basis for homework assignments that enable the client to practise skills that are relevant to goal achievement. In Sam's case, checking his fridge and pantry and noticing which essentials he has provides practice in attention and concentration. Creating a shopping list develops strategies for memory and assists with forward planning. When setting simple homework like this, check how well the client attended to the instructions. Explore strategies that will help them remember to do the homework (e.g. using mobile phone alarms).
- Monitor homework assignments. Success provides an encouraging indication of developing cognitive capacity. Failure provides an opportunity to more closely examine cognitive or motivational barriers to achievement.
- Work on tasks directly relevant to client goals. In Sam's case, job searching is directly relevant to his goals and requires several cognitive skills. Sam will need to work out a search strategy (planning) and, having identified potential sources of jobs, whether internet databases, newspaper advertisements or employment agency databases, will need to demonstrate effective attention and concentration to identify suitable jobs.
- Explain the connections between the cognitive exercises used in the cognitive remediation programme and the cognitive skills required for tasks that are central to client goals. As the programme develops, encourage the client to make these links independently.

How long should the training programme last?

There is no current research evidence to suggest the minimum or maximum number of sessions of brain training needed to obtain the best results. The various studies that have been conducted over the past 15 years range from as few as 16 sessions (Bellucci *et al.*, 2002) to beyond 12 months (Kurtz *et al.*, 2007). Also, the total time spent training can be well in excess of 100 hours (e.g. Bell *et al.*, 2008; Kurtz *et al.*, 2007) and the frequency of the training may involves sessions with the practitioner several times per week (Wykes *et al.*, 2007). At present, the best guide for clinical practice will be to sustain the remediation programme until the person has demonstrated improvements in their functioning in life domains that are important to them.

Summary

Cognitive problems of the type reported by Sam are common among people with severe mental illness. These problems often affect daily living and may be a major barrier to social inclusion through employment or other community activities. Cognitive remediation is a mental exercise programme that can be designed and implemented by a rehabilitation worker or case manager. The key tasks are assessing cognitive functioning, selecting cognitive exercises, maintaining motivation for regular cognitive exercise and building linkages between cognitive functioning and everyday activity. While cognitive remediation is reasonably demanding for both client and practitioner, the rewards and benefits are substantial because building cognitive capacity can provide a pathway to more independent living.

Acknowledgements

Drs Medalia, Keefe and Ventura are all warmly thanked for providing access to their measures.

Resources

Free online cognitive exercises:

http://playwithyourmind.com
http://cognitivefun.net

Some commercial providers of brain-training software:

http://www.psychological-software.com/psscogrehab.html
www.scilearnglobal.com
http://cognitiveenhancementtherapy.com

References

Altshuler L, Mintz J, Leight K (2002) The Life Functioning Questionnaire (LFQ): a brief, gender-neutral scale assessing functional outcome. *Psychiatry Research* **112**(2), 161–82.
Amador X, Strauss DH, Yale SA, Flaum MM, Endicott J, Gorman JM (1993) Assessment of insight in psychosis. *American Journal of Psychiatry* **150**, 873–9.
Bell MD, Zito W, Greig T, Wexler BE (2008) Neurocognitive enhancement therapy with vocational services: work outcomes at two-year follow-up. *Schizophrenia Research* **105**(1–3), 18–29.

Bellucci DM, Glaberman K, Haslam N (2002) Computer-assisted cognitive rehabilitation reduces negative symptoms in the severely mentally ill. *Schizophrenia Research* **59**, 225–32.

Birchwood M, Smith J, Cochrane R, Wetton S, Copestake S (1990) The Social Functioning Scale. The development and validation of a new scale of social adjustment for use in family intervention programmes with schizophrenic patients. *British Journal of Psychiatry* **157**(6), 853–9.

Bowie CR, Twamley EW, Anderson H, Halpern B, Patterson TL, Harvey PD (2007) Self-assessment of functional status in schizophrenia. *Journal of Psychiatric Research*, **41**(12), 1012–18.

Choi J, Mogami T, Medalia A (2010) Intrinsic Motivation Inventory: a scale adapted for schizophrenia research. *Schizophrenia Bulletin* **35**(5), 966–76.

Ehmann TS, Goldman R, Yager J, Xu Y, MacEwan GW (2007) Self-reported cognitive and everyday functioning in persons with psychosis: the Patient Perception of Functioning Scale. *Comprehensive Psychiatry* **48**(6), 597–604.

Grynszpan O, Perbal S, Pelissolo A *et al.* (2011) Efficacy and specificity of computer-assisted cognitive remediation in schizophrenia: a meta-analytical study. *Psychological Medicine* **41**, 163–73.

Heinrichs DW, Hanlon TE, Carpenter WT Jr (1984) The Quality of Life Scale: An instrument for rating the schizophrenic deficit syndrome. *Schizophrenia Bulletin* **10**(3), 388–98.

Keefe RSE, Poe M, Walker TM, Kang JW, Harvey PD (2006) The Schizophrenia Cognition Rating Scale: an interview-based assessment and its relationship to cognition, real-world functioning, and functional capacity. *American Journal of Psychiatry* **163**(3), 426–32.

Keefe RSE, Harvey PD, Goldberg TE *et al.* (2008) Norms and standardization of the Brief Assessment of Cognition in Schizophrenia (BACS). *Schizophrenia Research* **102**, 108–15.

Kurtz MM, Seltzer JC, Shagan DS, Thime WR, Wexler BE (2007) Computer-assisted cognitive remediation in schizophrenia: what is the active ingredient? *Schizophrenia Research* **89**(1–3), 251–60.

Leifker FR, Patterson TL, Heaton RK, Harvey PD (2011) Validating measures of real-world outcome: the results of the VALERO Expert Survey and RAND Panel. *Schizophrenia Bulletin* **37**, 334–43.

Lezak MD, Howieson DB, Loring DW (2004) *Neuropsychological Assessment*, 4th edn. Oxford University Press: New York.

Medalia A, Lim RW (2004) Self-awareness of cognitive functioning in schizophrenia. *Schizophrenia Research* **71**, 331–8.

Medalia A, Thysen J (2008) Insight into neurocognitive dysfunction in schizophrenia. *Schizophrenia Bulletin* **34**(6), 1221–30.

Ryan RM, Deci EL (2000) Self-determination theory and the facilitation of intrinsic motivation, social development, and well-being. *American Psychologist* **55**(1), 68–78.

Schneider LC, Struening EL (1983) SLOF: a behavioral rating scale for assessing the mentally ill. *Social Work Research and Abstracts* **19**(3), 9–21.

Stip E, Caron J, Renaud S, Pampoulova T, Lecomte Y (2003) Exploring cognitive complaints in schizophrenia: the subjective scale to investigate cognition in schizophrenia. *Comprehensive Psychiatry* **44**(4), 331–40.

Strauss E, Sherman EMS, Spreen O (2006) *A Compendium of Neuropsychological Tests*. Oxford University Press: New York.

Vansteenkiste M, Sheldon KM (2006) There's nothing more practical than a good theory: integrating motivational interviewing and self-determination theory. *British Journal of Clinical Psychology* **45**, 63–82.

Ventura J, Cienfuegos A, Boxer O, Bilder R (2008) Clinical global impression of cognition in schizophrenia (CGI-CogS): reliability and validity of a co-primary measure of cognition. *Schizophrenia Research* **106**(1), 59–69.

Wykes T, Huddy V (2009) Cognitive remediation for schizophrenia: it is even more complicated. *Current Opinion in Psychiatry* **22**(2), 161–7.

Wykes,T, Sturt E (1986) The measurement of social behaviour in psychiatric patients: an assessment of the reliability and validity of the SBS schedule. *British Journal of Psychiatry* **148**, 1–11.

Wykes T, van der Gaag M (2001) Is it time to develop a new cognitive therapy for psychosis – cognitive remediation therapy (CRT)? *Clinical Psychology Review* **21**, 1227–56.

Wykes T, Reeder C, Landau S *et al.* (2007) Cognitive remediation therapy in schizophrenia: randomised controlled trial. *British Journal of Psychiatry* **190**(5), 421–7.

Wykes T, Huddy V, Cellard C, McGurk SR, Czobor P (2011) A meta-analysis of cognitive remediation for schizophrenia: methodology and effect sizes. *American Journal of Psychiatry* **168**, 472–85.

Chapter 10

Treatment Adherence

Mitchell K. Byrne and Frank P. Deane

> Angela has been spending a fair bit of time with Sam in recent months. She is a 29-year-old single mother with one child. She studies part-time at the local university and has managed to maintain acceptable grades. She has bipolar disorder that has been well managed with medication, in different combinations at different points in her illness. However, over the last month she has intermittently missed doses and is consequently becoming unwell. It is puzzling that she is missing doses because she is very attached to her child and last time she stopped medication her daughter was placed in care. The following information was obtained from her in order to undertake a functional analysis.
>
> Financially, Angela was managing well on her supporting parent benefit and the maintenance paid by the father of her child. However, her former partner was sent to jail 3 months ago and the maintenance money he was sending her dried up. As a consequence, she started falling behind in some bills about 8 weeks ago. She has told you that this worries her. On top of this, her daughter started experiencing stomach aches last week and is cranky most of the time. Angela has said that she thinks that her daughter may be lactose intolerant and believes that her local GP did not take her concerns about her daughter's distress seriously enough when she took her to see him 10 days ago.
>
> Since becoming involved with Sam, Angela has struggled to keep a routine for her and her daughter and she says she forgets her medication from time to time. Sometimes Angela loses interest in sex and she thinks that her medication might reduce her libido.
>
> Angela has never received much help from her family because they don't agree with her diagnosis. He father says that she is just an attention getter and that she puts it on. He says that is why she cut herself when she was a teenager. Her father states that if she just stopped 'boozing' she wouldn't be so down and need the medication. Angela disagrees, stating that she has been drinking to help her sleep for years and is drinking no more or less now. Nonetheless, Angela has tried to cut down on her alcohol use over the last month and this has interfered with her sleep.

Introduction and key concepts

Severe mental health problems carry an enormous social and economic burden. Untreated, they usually worsen and result in a decline in the long-term prognosis (Burton, 2005). For many severe mental health problems, one of the most efficacious forms of treatment is pharmacotherapy, in particular the new 'atypical' antipsychotic medications (Gilmer *et al.*,

Manual of Psychosocial Rehabilitation, First Edition. Edited by Robert King, Chris Lloyd, Tom Meehan, Frank P. Deane and David J. Kavanagh.
© 2012 Blackwell Publishing Ltd. Published 2012 by Blackwell Publishing Ltd.

2004; Woltmann *et al.*, 2007). Effective management of major mental health disorders such as schizophrenia usually involves continuous long-term treatment in order to reduce the risk of relapse (Herz *et al.*, 1991). However, across all types of antipsychotic medication prescribed, non-adherence rates tend to be greater than 60% (Lieberman *et al.*, 2005).

The factors most consistently associated with non-adherence are poor insight, negative attitudes toward medication, previous non-adherence, substance abuse, shorter illness duration, inadequate discharge planning or aftercare environment, and poorer therapeutic alliance. Type of medication does not appear relevant (Lacro *et al.*, 2002). Idiosyncratic factors such as memory deficits (Elvevag *et al.*, 2003), cognitive difficulties with conceptualisation (Jeste *et al.*, 2003) and cultural factors, such as different illness representations (Opler *et al.*, 2004), need to be considered in order to understand an individual's non-adherence.

Such findings clearly suggest that non-adherence is determined by multiple factors (Happell *et al.*, 2002). Generally there are four categories which are used to capture the factors associated with treatment adherence:

- the treatment (e.g. complexity)
- the clinician (e.g. skill)
- the client (e.g. insight)
- the relationship between clinician and therapist (e.g. trust) (McDonald *et al.*, 2002; Meichenbaum & Turk, 1987; Zygmunt *et al.*, 2002).

Cognitive-behavioural therapies are among the most efficacious and comprehensive interventions to improve adherence. Cognitive-behavioural adherence interventions aim to get clients actively involved in their treatment and work collaboratively with clients to investigate the range of factors that might influence medication-taking behaviour (Gray *et al.*, 2002, 2010; Lecompte & Pelc, 1996). Cognitive and behavioural approaches form the basis of most contemporary adherence programmes such as motivational interviewing (Rollnick *et al.*, 2000; see Chapter 6), compliance therapy (Kemp *et al.*, 1996, 1998), medication management (Gray *et al.*, 2003, 2004), treatment adherence therapy (Staring *et al.*, 2010) and more recently, medication alliance (Byrne & Deane, 2011; Byrne *et al.*, 2004).

Adherence behaviour is rarely an 'all or nothing' affair (Sawyer & Aroni, 2003). Even partial non-adherence can have clinically significant effects upon the individual client (Weiden *et al.*, 2004). Any efforts to enhance adherence are likely to benefit the client. In the following sections we will explore some core strategies used to assist clients to effectively engage in treatment. We will emphasise the importance of establishing a strong *therapeutic* alliance with the client and the core intervention skill used to achieve this – *motivational interviewing* (see Chapter 6). While the focus will be on medications, these strategies should be considered 'transferable' across treatment domains, such as lifestyle issues, social relationships and other areas of psychosocial support provided to people with severe and enduring mental illness. The strategies, which have been drawn from the medication alliance programme, include:

- individualised assessment of medication-taking behaviour
- linking adherence to the client's goals

- assessing for and responding to the client's beliefs about treatment, including *normalising* non-adherence
- simplifying treatment and managing client impairments, such as deficits in executive functions, problem-solving skills deficits or dysfunctional beliefs.

We introduced Angela at the beginning of the chapter. Regular use of her mood-stabilising medication is critical to her mental health as well as to the wellbeing of her daughter. Angela is also a stabilising factor in Sam's life and if she becomes unstable, this will affect his mental health. How can Angela's rehabilitation practitioner work with her to improve her medication compliance?

Step 1: develop a hypothesis as to why Angela is experiencing difficulties with her medication at this time

The process of individualised assessment involves the identification of all possible causal variables contributing to the behaviour (non-adherence) and the collection of information about the relative contribution of these variables to the final behaviour (Haynes & Williams, 2003). Causal variables are identified by analysis of four core relationships between the proposed causal variable and the adherence behaviour. Haynes and colleagues (1997) state that a causal relationship exists between two variables when:

> (a) they co-vary (i.e. when one changes, so does the other), (b) the causal variable reliably precedes the dependent variable (i.e. the problem behaviour), (c) there is a logical connection, (d) alternative explanations for co-variance can be excluded. (p.334)

We can start our individualised assessment by looking at the information we have about events immediately surrounding the client's change in adherence behaviour. A useful tool in doing this is the ABC chart. The acronym 'ABC' stands for **A**ntecedents, **B**ehaviour and **C**onsequences. *Antecedents* refer to all the events or variables that preceded the client's changed behaviour; in the case of our example, this means changed medication-taking behaviour. *Behaviour* reflects the specifics of what the client is doing or has done in terms of their medication-taking behaviour. This means looking at how they are expressing their reduced adherence (*form*), ranging from mild resistance, expressions of dissatisfaction and being late to appointments through to complete refusal to use medication and discontinuation of treatment. Behaviour also looks at how long this has been happening (*duration*) and whether there are variations in this behaviour (*intensity*). Finally, *Consequences* refer to all the outcomes associated with the changed medication-taking behaviour, both positive and negative. Box 10.1 provides an example of the ABC approach for the 'Angela' vignette.

As you can see from Box 10.1, the 'Angela' vignette can be distilled into a series of key issues. When using the ABC approach, it is important to start with the behavior that you are interested in – the 'B'. In adherence interventions, this means we should always look at the medication-taking behaviour ('B') first, in order to understand exactly what the client is doing and when it started. The box identifies that the changes in behaviour began about 1 month ago. This is crucial information because it steers us away from more distant

---

Box 10.1 ABC analysis of 'Angela' vignette

Antecedents	Behaviour	Consequences
Loss of maintenance money 3 months ago	Misses doses intermittently	Reduced interest in boyfriend
Falling behind with bills 8 weeks ago	Has not discontinued all medication	Reduced libido
Daughter started having stomach aches a week ago	Began about a month ago and is escalating	Reduced mood
Poor alliance with GP (prescriber) 10 days ago		Sleep disturbance
New relationship began 6 weeks ago/change in routine		
Poor support from family (long term)		
Reduced use of alcohol resulting in reduced sleep for last month		
Reduced libido over last 2 weeks		

---

variables as causes of her changed behaviour. We also know that Angela has not stopped taking her medication altogether and that her pattern of medication use is variable. From this, we can hypothesise that she has not instigated a new regimen of medication use independently and that her reduced use of medication is probably not indicative of overall dissatisfaction with her treatment, although her reduced libido may either be a perceived side-effect influencing her adherence (an antecedent) or a result of her mood deterioration (a consequence).

An examination of the antecedents provides us with a lot of possible stressors or causes. Indeed, most clients are faced with frequent challenges, any one of which might precipitate a change in their medication-taking behaviour. How, then, do we 'rank' the possible causes according to their influence on behaviour? Generally speaking, *those events that occur closest to the change in behaviour are likely to be the most influential*. Using these guiding principles, we can generate a hypothesis about what is leading to or causing the medication non-adherence. Angela's medication-taking behaviour began to change about a month ago. Closely co-occurring events were the change in routine associated with her new relationship and poor sleep due to reduced alcohol use (and possibly exacerbated by her deteriorating mental health). Financial stress may have increased her vulnerability (see Step 3 below) and the issues with her daughter's health and her perceived relationship with her care provider/GP may have exacerbated her situation. However, changed routine and poor sleep appear to be the triggers for changed medication-taking behaviour.

Step 2: help Angela recognise patterns in the past and link these to Angela's goals

Often we find that clients cycle through patterns of adherence and non-adherence and that these may be predicted by life events. These life events are often useful in discovering, with the client, positive periods that have been associated with treatment adherence, and

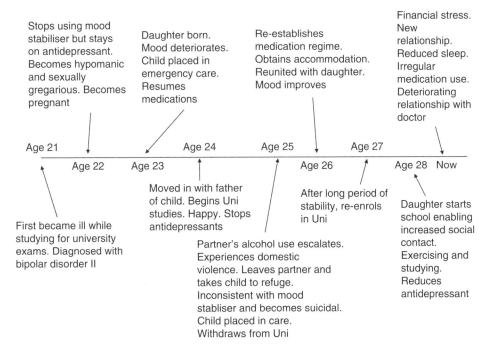

Stops using mood stabiliser but stays on antidepressant. Becomes hypomanic and sexually gregarious. Becomes pregnant

Daughter born. Mood deteriorates. Child placed in emergency care. Resumes medications

Re-establishes medication regime. Obtains accommodation. Reunited with daughter. Mood improves

Financial stress. New relationship. Reduced sleep. Irregular medication use. Deteriorating relationship with doctor

Age 21   Age 24   Age 25   Age 27

Age 22   Age 23   Age 26   Age 28   Now

First became ill while studying for university exams. Diagnosed with bipolar disorder II

Moved in with father of child. Begins Uni studies. Happy. Stops antidepressants

After long period of stability, re-enrols in Uni

Daughter starts school enabling increased social contact. Exercising and studying. Reduces antidepressant

Partner's alcohol use escalates. Experiences domestic violence. Leaves partner and takes child to refuge. Inconsistent with mood stabliser and becomes suicidal. Child placed in care. Withdraws from Uni

Figure 10.1   Angela's Illness Timeline.

negative experiences that have been associated with non-adherence. One tool that can facilitate this procress is called the Illness Timeline (Gray *et al.*, 2003). The Illness Timeline is like a diary of events in the individual's life, both positive and negative, and how those events have related to periods of health and ill health. Used in conjunction with the Stress/ Vulnerability Model (see below), the Illness Timeline enables both the practitioner and the client to organise and make sense of a wide range of information about the illness experience, including the relevance of adherence behaviours. It also enables the client to identify both 'positive' life experiences as well as experiences which they desired but have not been able to realise because of their illness. These 'desired experiences' may serve as intrinsic motivators to improve adherence behaviour. If adherence can be associated with the absence of negative experiences or the realisation of positive experiences, then motivation to adhere can be enhanced (see Chapter 6). Figure 10.1 provides an example of an Illness Timeline for Angela.

From Angela's Illness Timeline, we can see a pattern of stopping medication during periods of mental health, but a failure to reinstitute medication during times of stress. When Angela stops or reduces her medication and becomes unwell, she tends to lose contact with things she values in life, predominantly her daughter and her study. When Angela's mental health stabilises, she is able to re-establish her valued life goals. We can also see that establishing a medication routine during periods of stress is difficult for Angela. There is no personal history of difficulties associated with alcohol and so her father's comments (see vignette above) may not be accurate and require verification (although better strategies for sleep management should be considered).

The practitioner can combine the individualised assessment and the Illness Timeline to generate problem-solving strategies for the current difficulties as well as preventive plans for future problems that may be predicted from the Illness Timeline. The next step is to enhance Angela's understanding of her own adherence behaviours and to enable her to develop strategies to reduce her vulnerability to future relapse.

Step 3: link Angela's stressors and vulnerability

Life events are stressors that can predict ill health and the loss of valued life roles. Reducing vulnerability to these stressors can enhance desired life goals and act as an intrinsic motivator for treatment adherence. The Stress/Vulnerability Model emphasises that every individual varies across a number of illness-related dimensions, including genetic predispositions, physiological state, psychological characteristics and social engagement and support. Variations in these dimensions can affect the likelihood of a psychological breakdown. For example, a high biological vulnerability to illness means that fewer additional stressors, such as physical ill health or social isolation, are necessary before an individual may succumb to a psychotic event. Likewise, enhanced psychological health (e.g. through cognitive-behavioural therapy (CBT)), greater social and family support (e.g. through multiple-family groups) and enhanced physical health can reduce the likelihood that an otherwise vulnerable individual will experience an episode of mental ill health. The Stress/Vulnerability Model can be presented diagrammatically to clients as shown in Figure 10.2.

The diagram illustrates how lower levels of vulnerability to illness enable greater resilience to stressors, while higher vulnerability indicates that fewer stressors are needed to promote ill health. When using this with clients, the goal is to link strategies which

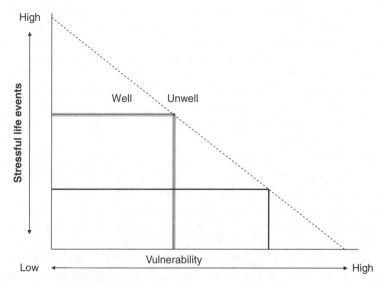

Figure 10.2   Simplified Stress/Vulnerability Model.

reduce vulnerability to the enhancement of resilience to day-to-day stressors. Of course, incorporating strategies to reduce stressors is also important.

Let's go back to the case study of Angela. We can see that financial stress placed Angela at increased risk of ill health. Angela was also stressed by increasing demands on her time through the new relationship and the health demands of her daughter. She is also stressed by the disruption to her sleep routine. In addition to her increased stress, Angela has reduced her medication. Medication acts to reduce her vulnerability and thus enhance her resilience. In essence, Angela has experienced a 'double whammy' of both increased stress and reduced resilience. This information might be used by the practitioner to help the client see the usefulness of both psychosocial interventions (to reduce stress) and medication adherence (to enhance resilience).

Step 4: normalise Angela's experiences and link changes to personally relevant goals

Mental ill health is fundamentally no different from other health conditions, although there may be more stigma associated with mental health problems. Often, it is the client themselves who holds this negative opinion and their resistance to treatment can be in part, a denial of their illness. The techniques described thus far can be applied to other health conditions and thus used as a means of destigmatising mental health.

To begin, it is important to explore with the client the notion that the brain is just another organ of the body: like the lungs, the heart or the liver, it can become unwell and may need treatment. Similarly, like other organs, environmental factors (e.g. stressors) can affect the health of the brain and medications can enhance the resilience of the brain (vulnerability).

We have found that using a simple example, such as high blood pressure, normalises the issues of mental ill health and the role of treatments such as medication (Figure 10.3). In this example, a person with a vulnerability to high blood pressure may experience

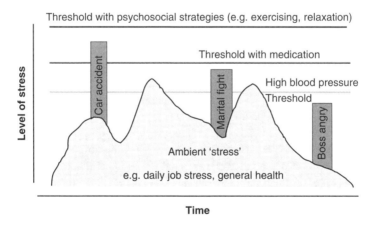

Figure 10.3   Example of Stress/Vulnerability Model using high blood pressure.

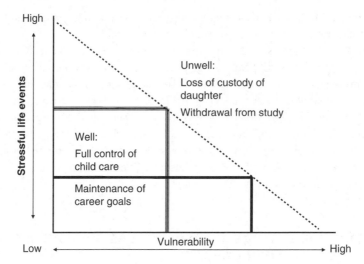

Figure 10.4   Angela's Stress/Vulnerability Model.

headaches and physical distress due to daily events (e.g. work-related demands) or because of major 'incidents' (e.g. a car accident). Their resilience to an elevation in blood pressure can be achieved through the use of medication and further enhanced with psychosocial interventions.

By using a normalising approach such as this, many clients are able to overcome resistance to treatment due to the perceived stigma of mental illness. However, resistance may be further reduced by identifying personally relevant goals from the Illness Timeline and mapping these onto the Stress/Vulnerability Model. For example, on Angela's Illness Timeline, it is clear that being well is associated with her ability to care for her daughter, while being unwell results in loss of custody. This can be shown to Angela in a simple stress/vulnerability diagram (Figure 10.4).

From time to time, clients may reject the idea that they have a mental illness at all, yet still observe that there are times in their life where desired goals were achieved and other times where events occurred that they would have preferred to avoid. Say, for example, that Angela denied her mental illness, yet she acknowledged losing custody of her daughter, accommodation and career goals (study). In this case, the vulnerability would refer not to mental ill health but rather to loss of independence or control over her life. By focusing on desired goals, she may associate the value of taking medication with more succesfully living independently. She may also associate non-adherence with the times when she was not adherent and lost her independence.

This 'discovery' can be created in a collaborative and non-threatening manner with the combined use of the Illness Timeline and Stress/Vulnerability Model. In this way, adherence is linked to a personally relevant goal (e.g. independence) and not to mental health or illness *per se*. Such an approach has similarities to motivational interviewing techniques where contemplation and decision preparation stages are met with decisional balance and scaling exercises. Refer to Chapter 6 for further information on motivational enhancement strategies.

Step 5: develop and implement an intervention that will work for Angela

Having agreed that enhancement in medication adherence is desirable, for reasons that match the client's motivations, the final step is to develop and implement a solution. Commonly this involves solving problems. Problem-solving techniques should be matched to the client's ability, with greater or lesser involvement of the practitioner depending on the client's degree of impairment. Impairments often experienced by people with significant mental health problems include comprehending, planning, paying attention, using or applying information, initiating or completing activities, using abstraction and remembering. These difficulties can affect a range of practical issues such as filling scripts, financial planning to pay for scripts, side-effect management, and lifestyle issues.

Generally speaking, irrespective of the level and type of impairment, the basic structure of problem-solving interventions is the same. The first stage of problem solving involves *defining the problem*. To define what the problem is, the following questions may be asked.

- What is the problem?
- Who is part of the problem?
- When does the problem occur?
- Where does the problem occur?
- What are the consequences of the problem?

In the case study of Angela, there are a number of problems. At this point it is worth remembering that some problems cannot be solved and thus must be accommodated. For example, Angela's previous partner cannot be released from prison before completion of his sentence. Furthermore, problems are often connected such that solving a 'higher order' problem can resolve subsequent issues arising from this problem. In Angela's case, her relationship and sexual difficulties may be problems arising from her deteriorating mental health, which itself is related to her reduced medication adherence. Thus the problem for Angela may simply be re-establishing a routine for medication.

The next step in problem solving is to restate the problem as a goal. This usually takes the form of 'to do such and such'. In Angela's case it might be as simple as 'to take my medication more consistently'. We then move from goals to solutions. At this point, the involvement of the client becomes critical as their investment in the solution will enhance the likelihood of a commitment to putting the solution into practice. Encouraging an array of possible solutions increases the likelihood that the client will collaboratively engage in the problem-solving process. Furthermore, encouraging wild or humorous possibilities facilitates engagement.

In Angela's situation, the following potential solutions may have arisen.

- Carry an alarm clock to remind me to take my medication.
- Get a dosette box.
- Ask my mum to ring me every night to remind me.
- Switch from an evening dose to a morning dose.

You may have thought of other potential solutions. At this point, each solution needs to be evaluated in terms of the positive and negative aspects associated with its implementation. In any case, the establishment of a routine that fits with Angela's current lifestyle would appear to be a key goal. While the issues of reduced libido, her daughter's ill health, financial stress and potential alcohol abuse remain, these may now be addressed with other psychosocial interventions.

Summary

Enhancing treatment adherence requires an individualised approach for each client. The value of adherence needs to be embedded in personally relevant goals or aspirations held by the client, which may include both the attainment and the avoidance of specific outcomes. Motivational interviewing strategies should be framed around individualised assessment, exploration of patterns of adherence across time (Illness Timeline), normalisation of illness and the logic of intervention (Stress/Vulnerability). The implementation of an adherence intervention should follow a process as outlined in Figure 10.5.

As outlined in Figure 10.5, any adherence intervention begins with an assumption that the client is at least ready to discuss their medication use. If this is not the case, the practitioner should engage in motivational interviewing strategies appropriate for 'Precontemplation' stages (as outlined in Chapter 6). Once some degree of ambivalence has been achieved, an individualised assessment of the specific *causal variables* associated with the client's changed adherence behaviour should be undertaken and linked to personally relevant life goals associated with previous adherence behaviours. This individualised assessment will identify a range of possible causes of non-adherence, including motivational issues, cognitive distortions, functional impediments (e.g. memory problems) or pragmatic issues. The practitioner is then in a position to target an intervention according to which of these causes of non-adherence is most relevant to the individual client.

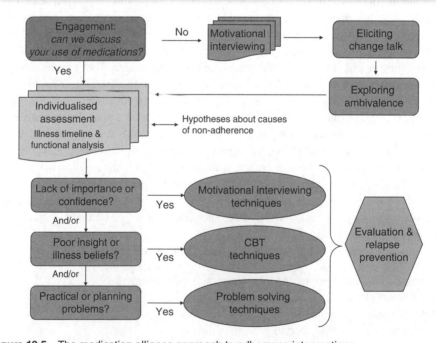

Figure 10.5   The medication alliance approach to adherence interventions.

References

Burton SC (2005) Strategies for improving adherence to second-generation antipsychotics in patients with schizophrenia by increasing ease of use. *Journal of Psychiatric Practice* **11**(6), 369–78.

Byrne MK, Deane FP (2011) Enhancing patient adherence: outcomes of medication alliance training on therapeutic alliance, insight, adherence and psychopathology with mental health patients. *International Journal of Mental Health Nursing* **20**(4), 284–95.

Byrne MK, Deane FD, Lambert G, Coombs T (2004) Enhancing medication adherence: clinician outcomes from the 'Medication Alliance' training program. *Australian and New Zealand Journal of Psychiatry* **38**, 246–53.

Elvevag B, Maylor EA, Gilbert AL (2003) Habitual prospective memory in schizophrenia. *BMC Psychiatry* **3**, 3–9.

Gilmer T, Dolder CR, Lacro JP *et al.* (2004) Adherence to treatment with antipsychotic medication and health care costs among Medicaid beneficiaries with schizophrenia. *American Journal of Psychiatry* **161**(4), 692–9.

Gray R, Wykes T, Gournay K (2002) From compliance to concordance: a review of the literature on interventions to enhance compliance with antipsychotic medication. *Journal of Psychiatric Mental Health Nursing* **9**(3), 277–84.

Gray R, Wykes T, Gournay K (2003) The effect of medication management training on community mental health nurse's clinical skills. *International Journal of Nursing Studies* **40**(2), 163–9.

Gray R, Wykes T, Edmonds M, Leese M, Gournay K (2004) Effect of a medication management training package for nurses on clinical outcomes for patients with schizophrenia: cluster randomised controlled trial. *British Journal of Psychiatry* **185**(2), 157–62.

Gray R, White J, Schulz M, Abderhalden C (2010) Enhancing medication adherence in people with schizophrenia: an international program of research. *International Journal of Mental Health Nursing* **19**, 36–44.

Happell B, Manias E, Pinikahana J (2002) The role of the inpatient mental health nurse in facilitating adherence to medication regimes. *International Journal of Mental Health Nursing* **11**, 251–9.

Haynes SN, Williams AE (2003) Case formulation and design of behavioral treatment programs: matching treatment mechanisms to causal variables for behavior problems. *European Journal of Psychological Assessment* **19**(3), 164–74.

Haynes SN, Leisen MB, Blaine DD (1997) Design of individualized behavioral treatment programs using functional analytic clinical case models. *Psychological Assessment* **9**(4), 334–48.

Herz MI, Glazer WM, Mostert MA *et al.* (1991) Intermittent vs. maintenance medication in schizophrenia. Two-year results. *Archives of General Psychiatry* **48**(4), 333–9.

Jeste SD, Patterson TL, Palmer BW, Dolder CR, Goldman S, Jeste DV (2003) Cognitive predictors of medication adherence among middle-aged and older outpatients with schizophrenia. *Schizophrenia Research* **63**(1–2), 49–58.

Kemp R, Hayward P, Applewhaite G, Everitt B, David A (1996) Compliance therapy in psychotic patients: randomised controlled trial. *British Medical Journal* **312**(7027), 345–9.

Kemp R, Kirov G, Everitt B, Hayward P, David A (1998) A randomised controlled trial of compliance therapy: 18-month follow-up. *British Journal of Psychiatry* **172**, 413–19.

Lacro JP, Dunn LB, Dolder CR, Leckband SG, Jeste DV (2002) Prevalence of and risk factors for medication nonadherence in patients with schizophrenia: a comprehensive review of recent literature. *Journal of Clinical Psychiatry* **63**(10), 892–909.

Lecompte D, Pelc I (1996) A cognitive-behavioural program to improve compliance with medication in patients with schizophrenia. *International Journal of Mental Health* **25**, 51–6.

Lieberman JA, Stroup TS, McEvoy JP *et al.* (2005) Effectiveness of antipsychotic drugs in patients with chronic schizophrenia. *New England Journal of Medicine* **353**(12), 1209–23.

McDonald HP, Garg AX, Haynes RB (2002) Interventions to enhance patient adherence to medication prescriptions. *Journal of the American Medical Association* **288**, 2868–79.

Meichenbaum D, Turk DC (1987) Treatment adherence: terminology, incidence and conceptualisation. In: Meichenbaum M, Turk D (eds) *Facilitating Treatment Adherence*. Plenum Press: New York, pp.19–39.

Opler LA, Ramirez PM, Dominguez LM, Fox MS, Johnson PB (2004) Rethinking medication prescribing practices in an inner-city Hispanic mental health clinic. *Journal of Psychiatric Practice* **10**(2), 134–40.

Rollnick S, Mason P, Butler C (2000) *Health Behavior Change: A Guide for Practitioners*. Churchill Livingstone: London.

Sawyer SM, Aroni RA (2003) Sticky issue of adherence. *Journal of Paediatric Child Health* **39**, 2–5.

Staring ABP, van der Caac M, Koopmans GT *et al*. (2010) Treatment adherence therapy in people with psychotic disorders: randomised controlled trial. *British Journal of Psychiatry* **197**, 448–55.

Weiden PJ, Kozma C, Grogg A, Locklear J (2004) Partial compliance and risk of rehospitalisation among Californian Medicaid patients with schizophrenia. *Psychiatric Services* **55**(8), 886–91.

Woltmann EM, Valenstein M, Welsh DE *et al*. (2007) Using pharmacy data on partial adherence to inform clinical care of patients with serious mental illness. *Psychiatric Services* **58**(6), 864–7.

Zygmunt A, Olfson M, Boyer CA, Mechanic D (2002) Interventions to improve medication adherence in schizophrenia. *American Journal of Psychiatry* **159**, 1653–64.

Part III
Reconnecting to the Community

Chapter 11

Social Skills and Employment

Philip Lee Williams and Chris Lloyd

Sam has been socialising less with friends and family members, choosing to stay in his room by himself for most of the day. Sam has stated that he used to enjoy spending time with friends but now finds this difficult because he doesn't feel he is able to communicate clearly. Sam would like to feel confident talking with people again and has set this as one of his goals as he feels that this will help him in finding and keeping work.

Bellack *et al.* (2004) define social skills as the 'interpersonal behaviours that are normative and/or socially sanctioned. They include such things as dress and behaviour codes, rules about what to say and not to say, and stylistic guidelines about the expression of affect, social reinforcement, interpersonal distance, and so forth' (p.3).

There are core skills (interactional skills, interpreting skills and responding and sending skills) used in this process, but a person's success in the application of these skills is determined by their ability to use them appropriately in specific social contexts. For this reason, Bellack *et al.* (2004) identify that whenever a professional provides social skills training, it is essential to be aware of the specific context in which the person wants to use those skills. Wherever possible, social skills training exercises, whether in a group or individual context, should be personalised to a specific situation in which a person would like to communicate more effectively.

As skills are developed, the next step is to develop a sense of confidence in the ability to transfer these skills to real-life situations. To achieve this, a person needs to develop a sense of mastery over these skills by applying them in simulated and safe real-life (such as with family or friends) situations. During this process it is useful to identify and celebrate any positive gains made while providing clear feedback about how to improve.

When considering the goals for treatment with a person, it is important to consider the stage of their illness, their premorbid social functioning (if relevant) and their individual goals for therapy. In general, people in the early stages of an illness are more likely to have more intact social skills than someone with a longer history.

Manual of Psychosocial Rehabilitation, First Edition. Edited by Robert King, Chris Lloyd, Tom Meehan, Frank P. Deane and David J. Kavanagh.
© 2012 Blackwell Publishing Ltd. Published 2012 by Blackwell Publishing Ltd.

Once the goal of improving social skills has been identified by the person, the process of engaging and addressing the issues are the same as with any other treatment goal. Start by completing an assessment of the person's current social functioning and identify their specific goals for therapy. The goal attainment scale (GAS see below) offers a useful tool to identify specific, measurable consumer goals. Importantly this tool gives the therapist and consumer the opportunity to clearly record and evaluate the desired outcomes from participating in therapy. Following this process consider the most appropriate intervention method (group or individual) to develop the required skills and/or confidence. Provide the intervention and evaluate the treatment outcomes. It is always useful to have one maintenance/follow up session after the evaluation session to review the application of the skills learnt.

In the example provided above, the initial step is to accurately determine which social skills and in what contexts Sam feels most and least confident, negotiating which context he would like to work on most. A useful framework you might like to use to guide this process is the brief solution focused therapy framework (see below) discussed by George *et al.* (1990) and Sharry *et al.* (2001).

Useful topics to explore with Sam

*   In what contexts is Sam most likely to be using his social skills – at home, with friends, looking for work?
*   In which contexts does Sam feel most confident and least confident?
*   Which social context does Sam want to work on most?
*   Is Sam confident in initiating, maintaining and ending a conversation?
*   How confident is Sam following conversations with people he knows well and/or strangers?
*   Does Sam feel he can accurately read the emotional expressions of people he knows well? Does Sam feel he can accurately read the emotional expressions of people he does not know?
*   Is Sam confident in being assertive when he would like to be?
*   What are the specific skills required for the context you are working on with Sam?

A desire to return to work is a common goal, particularly for those in the early stages of an illness. In order to achieve this, addressing social functioning specifically related to the work setting is important. The Work Related Self-Efficacy Scale (Waghorn *et al.*, 2005), described below, could be used for this. Items pertaining to work-related social skills include: co-operate closely with people helping you prepare for work, use your social network to identify job opportunities, ask an employer (in person or by telephone) for information about a job, participate appropriately in a job interview, ask relevant questions during a job interview, request urgent leave from the supervisor, check instructions with the supervisor, decline a request to work overtime, request a change of hours or days of working, resolve a conflict with a colleague, resolve a conflict with a superior, decline a request to exchange duties of work days, help to instruct or demonstrate a task to a new colleague, co-operate with other workers to perform a group task, and follow directions without resistance.

For Sam, in addition to the core social skills, you should explore work-related social skills.

- How confident is Sam about participating in interviews?
- How confident is Sam about negotiating common workplace interactions, e.g. shift times, days off, overtime, holidays?
- How confident is Sam in meeting the dress and personal presentation standards of the workplace?
- Can Sam confidently discuss work-related tasks with his supervisor, e.g. seeking help with tasks, checking instructions?
- How confident is Sam when negotiating job tasks with co-workers, e.g. seeking help, delegating tasks, taking instructions?
- Are there social skill requirements that are specific to Sam's workplace?
- Does Sam want to/feel comfortable disclosing his mental illness with his boss?

Useful tools and resources for social skills training

As with all other assessments, it is important to have a clear reason (e.g. relates to a specific goal) for completing an assessment with a person.

Assessments

- The Adaptive Behaviour Assessment Scale (ABAS) is a standardised questionnaire which is a useful tool for assessing a person's general adaptive skills and includes a specific item relating to social skills. It provides an overall awareness of a person's functioning. Three domains of adaptive behaviour are assessed: conceptual skills, social skills and practical skills. The ABAS takes approximately 45 minutes to complete.
- Another tool which is particularly useful is the Work-Related Self-Efficacy Scale (WSS-37) (Waghorn *et al.*, 2005). This 37-item scale measures self-efficacy in four relevant activity domains: vocational service access and career planning, job acquisition, work-related social skills, and general work skills. The WSS-37 was developed in a 12-month longitudinal survey of people diagnosed with schizophrenia or schizoaffective disorder. The results from this indicated validity of both a four-factor structure differentiating four core skill domains and a single factor representing total work-related self-efficacy. The WSES-37 is a self-report measure with confidence rated on an 11-point scale (from 0 = no confidence to 100 = total confidence) (Waghorn *et al.*, 2007). Harris *et al.* (2010) reported on the WSS-37 reliability and validity with individuals with schizophrenia and schizoaffective disorder and recommended its use in supported education programmes.
- The brief solution focused therapy approach focuses on what clients want to achieve through therapy rather than on their problems. George *et al.* (1990) outline a number of techniques that can be used in therapy that guides clients down this path. Examples of these tools include the 'miracle question' which asks clients to describe, in detail, what their life will be like when all their problems have gone, scaling questions, exception-seeking questions and coping questions. A key to this approach is agreeing with the client to keep the discussion in each session 'problem free'.

- It is recommended that if you have not already done so, you consider the presence of co-morbidities such as anxiety or depression, which may significantly affect a person's social skills. The Depression Anxiety Stress Scale (DASS) is a useful screening tool for this (Lovibond & Lovibond, 1995).
- The Goal Attainment Scale (GAS) is a useful tool to track the progress Sam makes as he engages in therapy (Kiresuk & Sherman, 1968; Lloyd, 1986). The GAS is a five-point scale created by an individual with the support of a practitioner to record the potential outcomes for a goal (see Tables 11.1 and 11.2). This scale provides an indicator for overachieving and underachieving for a goal and a method for measuring the degree of success in achieving the goal. Once a goal has been identified with a client, the practitioner should discuss how they would now feel if they achieved more than they hoped or less than they hoped before recording this as shown in Table 11.2.

Table 11.1   Goal Attainment Scale.

Score	Description
+ 2	Most favourable outcome
+ 1	More than expected outcome
0	Expected outcome
– 1	Less than expected outcome
– 2	Much less than expected outcome

Table 11.2   Example of Goal Attainment Scale.

Goal	'I will be able to confidently approach a business and hand in my resumé when looking for a job'	'I will be able to participate in a job interview'
Most favourable outcome +2	Sam will be able to hand in his resumé and have a short conversation with the employer on his skills and abilities and follow up the conversation 2 days later with a phone call	Sam will be able to independently and confidently participate in a job interview, being able to answer all the questions, feel relaxed and positively sell his skills for the job
More than expected outcome +1	Sam will be able to hand in his resumé and have a short conversation about his skills	Sam will be able to answer the questions required in a job interview and use the questions to sell all his skills
Expected outcome 0	Sam will be able to independently organise time to go job searching and will be able to walk into a business, introduce himself and hand over his resumé	Sam will be able to answer the questions required in a job interview
Less than expected outcome – 1	Sam will be able to hand in his resumé at the front counter	Sam will be able to attend a job interview but might struggle to answer some of the questions
Most unfavourable outcome –2	Sam will not be able to approach a business to hand in his resumé without support	Sam won't be able to attend a job interview

Resources

There are scores of resources available relating to this area but the following provide a good starting point.

- Bellack *et al.* (2004) is a useful detailed text outlining treatment approaches for social skills training in schizophrenia.
- Kingsep and Nathan (ND) have produced a useful and detailed treatment manual for group therapy through the Western Australian Department of Health Centre for Clinical Interventions.
- The US Department of Veterans Affairs has some useful training video clips that can be accessed without cost from their website at: http://www.mirecc.va.gov/visn5/training/sst/section1/sst_video_section1.asp.

Sam has reported that he used to be an outgoing person who was seen by others as somebody who was fun to be around. Since becoming unwell, he has found himself more withdrawn and finds it hard to talk with other people. During assessment, Sam reports that he is embarrassed by his lack of ability to talk with people and that this is one of the reasons he avoids his friends and has avoided seeking employment. Sam is not sure if he will be able to improve his social skills and is worried that this is part of the illness that he will have to live with. Although Sam is unsure if he will be able to improve his confidence in social interactions in the work environment, he has agreed to work on them in sessions with the practitioner.

It is decided that a group programme is the best avenue for Sam to practise and gain confidence using social skills he will need in the workplace. From the assessment, however, it is evident that Sam finds group situations where he is required to socialise very difficult at present. Sam agrees to practise core communication skills with a practitioner to improve his confidence before attending the group.

Individual sessions

Session 1

Conversation starters

Develop phrases that Sam could use for each topic when in conversation with someone. Sam should write these phrases down before practising them in a role-play situation with the practitioner. Some examples might include, for someone who is known: 'Hi, how's it going?' or 'Hello, I haven't seen you for a while. What have you been up to?'; for someone who is unknown, this might be: 'Hello, my name is Sam, what's your name?'.

Dealing with difficult questions

Discuss and plan phrases that Sam could use to answer questions that might be uncomfortable. An example might include Sam being asked by another group member to share personal information about his diagnosis and treatment; he might respond with a general answer and redirect the conversation using a question: 'It's still up in the air – hey, did you see the … last night on TV/news?'.

Session 2

Maintaining a conversation

Discuss and practise techniques that Sam could use to keep a conversation going, for example, active listening skills, using open-ended questions, how to make chit-chat using neutral topics like the weather or recent activities.

Finishing a conversation

Discuss and practise socially acceptable ways in which Sam could end a conversation if he wanted to, for example, looking at his watch before making an excuse that he had to be somewhere or by saying: 'thanks for saying hello, do you mind if I go and catch some of the other people?'

Session 3

Reading body language

Use popular magazines or films (with the sound muted) to identify the emotions displayed in the person's body language. It is good to start with films like comedies or sit-coms where emotions are overacted before moving on to scenes from dramas.

> After completing three sessions with the practitioner, Sam feels able to try attending a group programme. He remains ambivalent about his ability to interact with other group members but is willing to have a go.

A social skills group programme: talking shop

Outline

The aim of this group programme is to establish a safe environment which encourages group participants to learn, practise and use social skills. In the example below, each session is focused around an activity that all group members can participate in. As the example below is for Sam, the activity sessions will be sports based. Depending on the group cohort any team based activity would be suitable for this group (see Box 11.1).

Standard session plan

- Warm-up activity (Table 11.3)
- Review homework
- First half – activity (Box 11.1)
- Break from activity – education session
- Second half – activity
- Cooldown and wrap-up (Table 11.4) – finish activity and summarise education session

Table 11.3   Warm-up activities.

Name	Process
My shoes	Get each group member to describe their shoes and tell one story about where their shoes have been
What type of biscuit/animal/flower are you?	Get each group member to describe what type of biscuit/animal/flower they would be and describe why
Finish the sentence	Get each person in the group to finish one of three sentences: 'The best holiday I have had is …' 'The best job I have had is …' 'The best concert I have been to is …'
Marooned	Each member tells the group what would be the five things they would take if they were marooned on an island
Find the lie	Give each participant a piece of paper and a pen. Get each person to write three things about themselves – two things that are true and one that is false. The group has to choose which item is false

---

Box 11.1   Group activity options

Tennis	Knitting
Basketball	Art
Volleyball	Sewing
Table tennis	Pottery
Gym	Gardening
Walking: beach, local park or forest park	Surfing
Tai chi	Cooking
Scrabble	Card making/scrap booking

Table 11.4   Cooldown/wrap-up options.

Option	Process
Sporting/active activity	• Complete a short task as a group, e.g. one lap of a basketball court • Group facilitator to lead 5 minutes of gentle stretching for each of the major muscle groups: calves, hamstrings, abdominals/back, chest, shoulders and neck. Finish with a brief deep breathing exercise • Each person to tell the group one thing they will take home from the group today
Non-sporting activity	• Complete a 5-minute guided relaxation exercise, e.g. observe your breath, guided imagery or scanning exercise to help prepare people for leaving the group • Each person to tell the group one thing they will take home from the group today

Tip: Discuss with the group whether they would like to choose one activity such as tennis or basketball for the whole group programme or try a different activity each week. The activity chosen for the group needs to match the skills, abilities, interests and age of the participants. Access to the appropriate resources to run the activity also needs to be considered.

Tip: If possible, it is useful for a practitioner/case manager to meet with Sam after each weekly session to discuss his experience in the group session and reinforce the education sessions.

Session 1: Introduction

Purpose: introduce group members to each other and confirm the goals of the group.

- Introduction: explain the purpose of the group programme, its duration and the expected topics for each session. It is important to establish the group rules and plan the activity sessions during this initial meeting.
- Warm-up: finish the sentence (Table 11.3).
- Group expectations: discuss why members have chosen to attend this group programme. These can be brainstormed as a group. Invite members to write two goals they would like to achieve by attending the group. Write these goals using the Goal Attainment Scale format.
- Group programme
  - Explain the format of the group programme. Decide as a group which activities will be completed each week. It is useful to provide the group with a list of possible activities.
  - General group rules that should be discussed include: maintaining confidentiality, commitment to the group, maintaining respect for fellow group members, arriving on time, phoning if unable to attend, completing homework tasks.
- Activity: finish with a group activity. The chosen activity should be something appropriate for the skills and abilities of the group members and should include some aspect of communication, e.g. volleyball, tenpin bowling, Wii competition, group Pictionary, plan a gardening activity.
- Cooldown and wrap-up (Table 11.4).

Session 2: The nuts and bolts of communication

- Warm-up: 'My shoes' (Table 11.3).
- Activity: basketball.
- Break from activity – education session.
  - Discuss the role of body language in communication. A simple activity is to get group members to work in pairs with one person displaying an emotion with facial expressions only and the other person guessing what emotion it is.
  - Discuss the communication process, including the role of the giver (their thoughts, body language and words), the message (what is said) and the receiver (their thoughts, body language and words).
  - Discuss simple conversation starters, maintainers and finishers. Each person should write down the phrases they would use and share them with the group.
  - Role play: working in pairs, each person is given a social situation to role play. Social situations can include 'Meeting an old school friend at an informal function', 'Meeting a colleague outside work'.
  - Homework: each participant should plan three situations in which they can practise these basic communication skills, e.g. with family, with a person at the supermarket checkout.
- Cooldown and wrap-up (Table 11.4).

Session 3: Effective communication – saying what you want to and being heard

- Warm-up: 'Marooned' (Table 11.3).
- Review: review homework task from previous week and any questions group members may have.
- Activity: basketball.
- Break from activity – education session.
  - Discuss strategies, such as planning, that can be used to help group participants ensure they remember to say what they want to, e.g. Use a list
  - Discuss techniques participants can use to check if someone has understood their message correctly, e.g. Asking for statements to be repeated
  - Discuss strategies that participants can use to clarify their message if they haven't been heard correctly, e.g. Re-wording statement
  - Use a popular TV series to highlight examples of good communication and poor communication for the group to critique.
  - Homework: participants should identify one situation where they have had difficulty communicating to practise these new strategies, e.g. Discussing treatment plan with your doctor
- Cooldown and wrap-up (Table 11.4).

Session 4: Assertiveness

- Warm-up: what type of biscuit/animal/flower are you? (Table 11.3)
- Review: review homework task from previous week and any questions group members may have.
- Activity: basketball.
- Break from activity – education session.
  - Discuss the three major communication styles: passive, assertive and aggressive (including passive aggressive). Discuss phrases and strategies people can use to be assertive in their communication styles.
  - Role play: group members to identify assertive phrases that they would feel comfortable using and practise these in pairs.
  - Homework: provide group members with a list of possible everyday scenarios in which they can practise their assertiveness skills, e.g. negotiating medical appointment times, negotiating shared household tasks such as cleaning duties, returning wrong orders at a café, negotiating treatment plans. Group members are to practise their skills in one of these situations.
- Cooldown and wrap-up. (Table 11.4)

Session 5: Break in education

- Warm-up: 'Find the lie' (Table 11.3).
- Review: review homework task from previous week and any questions group members may have.
- Activity: basketball.

- Break from activity – revision.
  - Summarise the previous three education sessions.
  - Lead the group in a discussion about how they have applied any of the skills from each education session. Ensure that you explore any difficulties group members may have had when applying the skills learnt in the group in the real world and celebrate any success that group members have had.
  - In groups of three, get group members to role play common social interactions using the skills they have learnt. By this stage it should be possible to get the group to identify up to four social situations for the role plays. If they cannot, you might like to use: meeting a new friend for coffee at a local café, negotiating a new treatment plan with your doctor, telling your boss of a problem in the workplace.
- Cooldown and wrap-up (Table 11.4).

Session 6: Getting ready for work – job interview skills

- Warm-up: for the second half of the programme, you can either use the above warm-up activities again or ask one group member a week to bring a warm-up activity of their own.
- Activity: indoor football (utilising the same venue as used for basketball).
- Break from activity – education session.
  - Discuss the process of a job interview.
  - Discuss helpful tips to prepare for a job interview such as planning your route to arrive on time, arriving at least 15 minutes early, dressing appropriately for the interview.
  - Discuss the role of body language in a job interview.
  - Discuss and role play introducing yourself to the interviewer.
  - Discuss and role play answering questions from the interviewer individually with the facilitator.
  - Homework: locate a video on the internet that shows how to do a job interview.
- Cooldown and wrap-up (Table 11.4).

Session 7: Communicating with your supervisor

- Warm-up.
- Review: review homework task from previous week and any questions group members may have.
- Activity: indoor football.
- Break from activity – education session.
  - Use video excerpts from 'The Office' or a similar popular TV show or movie as stimulus to discuss the following.
  - Discuss participants' experience of communicating with supervisors. Identify the similarities and differences with communicating with a friend.
  - Discuss strategies for clarifying information given by the supervisor.
  - Discuss strategies for communicating requests, such as taking leave, with the supervisor.

○ Optional task: discuss how clients should interact with their supervisor if they become unwell.
- Cooldown and wrap-up (Table 11.4).

Session 8: How to handle conflict and find solutions for difficult problems

- Warm-up.
- Review: review homework task from previous week and any questions group members may have.
- Activity: indoor football.
- Break from activity – education session.
  ○ Discuss problem-solving strategies and work through a group problem-solving activity.
  ○ Discuss how conflict in the workplace can arise. The role of simple communication errors should be emphasised (use a video example from a film or popular TV show such as 'The Office').
  ○ Discuss principles to address workplace conflict including approaching the person, negotiating and compromising. Model addressing a workplace conflict such as your colleague works with the radio on all day and you want it turned off sometimes.
  ○ Discuss how and when to discuss issues with the supervisor. Get the group to brainstorm strategies for approaching a supervisor, e.g. negotiate a time to meet with the supervisor, write down your points and your preferred outcome prior to the meeting.
- Cooldown and wrap-up (Table 11.4).

Session 9: Putting it all together

- Warm-up.
- Activity: indoor football.
- Break from activity – education session.
  ○ Revise the previous three education sessions with group participants.
  ○ Summarise the basic communication skills discussed in the first 5 weeks and link them to the specific work-related social skills in the second half of the programme.
  ○ Group participants should discuss and write down how they will use the skills and confidence gained from the programme.
  ○ Review group participants' goals (written using the Goal Attainment Scale) developed in the beginning of the programme.
  ○ Complete group programme evaluation.
- Cooldown and wrap-up (Table 11.4).

Session 10: Celebration

- Activity: this week is about using the skills learnt during the group programme by participating in a group celebration activity. The activity will vary depending on the group composition but could possibly include an outing to a restaurant or café, a BBQ or picnic, a special activity to be organised by the group such as surfing classes or indoor rock climbing.

○ Use newfound skills to share with the group a positive experience stemming from the group programme.

○ Share one skill that they need to work on.

Sam has completed the group programme and has identified that he feels more confident engaging in social situations. He has been actively seeking employment during the course of the programme and is looking forward to obtaining work. While he continues to look for work, Sam has set himself a goal of keeping in regular contact with friends and continuing to attend an activity group to maintain the confidence he has gained from the programme.

Sam is highly motivated to return to work but has been struggling to complete the required tasks to successfully gain employment. He has agreed to focus on skills that will assist him to obtain employment with his case manager.

Tip: Where possible it is useful to complete both the return to work activities and social skills activities at the same time.

Employment

There are many models that can be used to plan effective vocational rehabilitation services. As always, the needs of the client must be considered in conjunction with the resources available to the case manager and service. Examples of effective vocational rehabilitation models include supported employment (also known as the IPS (Individual Placement and Support) Model); job networks; clubhouse; social firms and business services (sheltered workshops). A useful description of these models can be found in Waghorn and Lloyd (2005).

The IPS Model is currently considered best practice in establishing and providing vocational rehabilitation services for people living with a mental illness and has consistently demonstrated promising results across multiple randomised controlled trials (Waghorn and Lloyd, 2005). Drake and Becker (1996) describe the seven key principles of the IPS Model (see below). Overarching these seven key principles is the shift away from the traditional 'train then place' approach to vocational rehabilitation to a new 'place then train' approach (Tsang, 2008).

The IPS model consists of seven key principles (Drake and Becker, 1996; Waghorn and Lloyd, 2005).

- Eligibility is based on client choice.
- Integration of vocational rehabilitation services with mental health services.
- Competitive employment is the goal.
- Rapid commencement of job search activities.
- Services based on client preferences.
- Continuing support to retain employment.
- Income support and health benefits counselling.

Tsang (2008) has demonstrated that integrating social skills training with the IPS Model enhances success rates for people seeking employment. Where possible to do so, this is recommended.

The role of the service

Where it is possible to establish the IPS Model, the role of the case manager is to support the client to engage with the employment specialist and maintain regular communication between the client, employment specialist and mental health service. Much of the work described below will be completed by the employment/vocational rehabilitation specialist in this situation. Without labouring the point too much, one of the critical components to the success of this model is the development and maintenance of time where the employment worker and case manager work alongside each other in the same space, allowing effective communication to occur.

If the required components are not in place to support the IPS Model, it is recommended that practitioners focus on providing individual (or if possible group-based) support to the clients wanting to re-enter the job market.

> Sam is completing the social skills programme and has said that he feels ready to return to the workforce. There are no specialised employment support agencies that Sam can be referred to. Sam has agreed to complete individual sessions focusing on the steps required to return to the workforce.
>
> Sam agrees to attend individual sessions once a week with the case manager at the clinic.

Individual sessions

Session 1: Resumé writing

Ask the client to bring along a copy of their old resumé. If they don't have one, it would be useful to have available a template of a resumé that they can use to create one. To best support the client in finishing their resumé, it is ideal to have access to a computer that they can use to complete the resumé. Alternatively, you may like to get them to hand write the resumé and then type it up later. The homework task is for the client to have completed the resumé by the next scheduled session.

Session 2: Job search strategies

- Discuss what methods of job searching the client has used before. It is best to focus on the strategies that have worked well for people in the past. You may also like to cover the following.
  - Newspapers: on which day are the jobs advertised and which newspapers are best for the jobs they are seeking?
  - Recruitment agencies: are there any job recruitment agencies in the local area that the client could access and what is the referral process?

○ Online searches: demonstrate how to search for jobs using the internet. It would be advisable to identify these prior to the session.
○ Walk-ins: discuss the advantages/disadvantages to walking into businesses off the street and providing your resumé.
- Making the enquiry call: role play calling up a business in response to a job advertisement to seek more information. It would be helpful to get the client to write down what they should say after the first practice go.

Session 3: The interview

Interviews are difficult for most people. Before moving into role playing an interview, consider the context in which the interview is most likely to occur, e.g. formal panel, informal talk with the boss, multiple interview techniques? Once this is identified discuss the following.

- What you should do to prepare for the interview.
- How you should dress.
- How to manage your nerves in the interview, e.g. distraction techniques like squeezing your hands.
- How to make sure you get there on time – planning your route.
- Questions you would like to ask.

Practise the interview in a role-play situation until the client feels comfortable answering the questions. Plenty of positive reinforcement should be used here.

Session 4: Deciding on disclosure

Depending on the client's insight, this session can either be run as the first session or later, as is presented here.

   Deciding to disclose to an employer about your mental health history is a big deal and should be a decision the client makes for themselves. If an employment specialist is available, this process can be supported by them. There are benefits and disadvantages on both sides when considering disclosing. If the consumer decides to disclose, discuss specifically what information they would like disclosed and how they would like this to happen.

Session 5: Maintaining employment

- Social supports play a key role in giving a person the ongoing support required to maintain employment. Discuss who the client feels are key social supports for them and how they plan to maintain contact with these people.
- Managing stress is essential.
   ○ Review/teach relaxation strategies including using relaxation exercises, engaging in weekly leisure activities and using your leave effectively to decrease stressors when required.
   ○ Review/develop the relapse prevention plan for the client.

Tip: These sessions can either be run individually or if there are sufficient numbers to form a group, can be run in a group situation using the same structure as described above.

Summary

This chapter has provided a guide to the process of addressing social skills and employment using group and individual programmes with a client. Social skills training has been a core aspect of mental health treatment for many years and as a result there are numerous resources available for both individual and group programmes.

Where available, it is highly recommended that an Individual Placement and Support Model of vocational rehabilitation be established. However, if this is not available then engaging the client in active job seeking when they are motivated to return to the workforce in conjunction with individual/group support provides the best chance of a successful return to the workforce.

References

Bellack AS, Mueser KT, Gingerich S, Agresta J (2004) *Social Skills Training in Schizophrenia: A Step By Step Guide*. Guilford Press: New York.

Drake RE, Becker DR (1996) The individual placement and support model of supported employment. *Psychiatric Services* **47**, 473–5.

George E, Iveson C, Ratner H (1990) *Problem to Solution: Brief Therapy with Individuals and Families*. BT Press: London.

Harris M, Gladman B, Hennessy N, Lloyd C, Mowry B, Waghorn G (2010) Reliability of a scale of work-related self-efficacy for people with psychiatric disabilities. *International Journal of Rehabilitation Research* **33**(2), 183–6.

Kingsep P, Nathan P (ND) *Social Skills Training for Severe Mental Disorders: A Therapist Manual*. Western Australian Department of Health, Centre for Clinical Interventions. www.cci.health.wa.gov.au/resources/minipax.cfm?mini_ID=18

Kiresuk TJ, Sherman R (1968) Goal attainment scaling: a general method for evaluating comprehensive community mental health programs. *Community Mental Health Journal* **4**, 443–53.

Lloyd C (1986) The process of goal setting using goal attainment scaling in a therapeutic community. *Occupational Therapy in Mental Health* **6**(3), 19–30.

Lovibond P, Lovibond S (1995) The structure of negative emotional states comparison of the Depression Anxiety Stress Scales (DASS) with the Beck Depression and Anxiety Inventories. *Behaviour Research and Therapy* **33**(3), 335–43.

Sharry J, Madden B, Darmody M (2001) *Becoming a Solution Detective. A Strengths-Based Guide to Brief Therapy*. BT Press: London.

Tsang H (2008) Enhancing employment opportunities of people with mental illness through an integrated supported employment approach of individual placement and support and social skills training. *Hong Kong Medical Journal* **14**(3), 41–6.

Waghorn G, Lloyd C (2005) The employment of people with a mental illness. *Australian e-Journal for the Advancement of Mental Health* **4**(2), 1–43.

Waghorn G, Chant D, King R (2005) Work-related self-efficacy among community residents with psychiatric disabilities. *Psychiatric Rehabilitation Journal* **29**(2), 105–13.

Waghorn G, Chant D, King R (2007) Work-related subjective experiences, work-related self-efficacy, and career learning among people with psychiatric disabilities. *American Journal of Psychiatric Rehabilitation* **10**, 275–300.

Chapter 12

Healthy Lifestyles

Chris Lloyd and Hazel Bassett

> Sam has been drinking too much. He has been feeling bored. He has put on some weight since he has been sitting around not knowing what to do with his time. Sam has been a bit worried about how he has been feeling and has decided that he needs to do something about it.

As Sam's case manager or rehabilitation practitioner, how can you help him?

Step 1: Start with an assessment of Sam (Table 12.1)

This would probably be best in the form of a semi-structured interview plus the use of some standardised assessments. You will need to address the following.

Substance use

- How much has he been drinking?
- When does he drink?
- What was he doing prior to drinking?
- Why does he think he drinks?
- How long has he been drinking?
- Has he committed any offences while intoxicated?
- Has he had any withdrawal symptoms?
- Does he think that his substance use is out of control?
- Is he worried about his substance use?
- Does he wish he could stop?
- How difficult would he find it to go without?
- Does he want to change his substance use right now?
- Does he think he could change his use of substances now if he wanted to?

If you want to assess his readiness to change, the Readiness to Change questionnaire (Rollnick *et al.*, 1992) may be useful.

Manual of Psychosocial Rehabilitation, First Edition. Edited by Robert King, Chris Lloyd, Tom Meehan, Frank P. Deane and David J. Kavanagh.
© 2012 Blackwell Publishing Ltd. Published 2012 by Blackwell Publishing Ltd.

Table 12.1   Assessment tools for substance use.

Title	Description	Use
Alcohol Use Disorders Identification Test screening instrument (AUDIT: Sanders *et al.*, 1993)	Ten items measuring three domains: alcohol consumption, alcohol dependence, alcohol-related consequences. Takes 2–5 minutes to complete	Screening instrument. Suitable to use with a wide range of cultures. Can be used with people with a minimum reading level
Short Alcohol Dependence Data questionnaire (SADD: Raistrick *et al.*, 1983)	Fifteen items measuring severity of dependence on alcohol; reflects behaviour and subjective change associated with problem drinking. Takes less than 5 minutes to complete	Instrument to measure severity of alcohol dependence. Suitable for use with a range of ethnic groups and cultures. Can be used in an interview format with illiterate populations

Diet

- What is his daily intake of food like?
- Does he eat three meals per day?
- Is he prone to eating snacks?
- What sort of snacks does he eat?
- Does he know how to cook?
- Does he do the cooking or is it done for him?
- If he cooks, what sorts of things does he cook?
- Is he wanting to know more about nutrition?
- Is he wanting assistance with meal planning and preparation?
- Can he identify times when he overeats?

If you want to measure food intake and to also note possible mood effects on the intake of food, then a food/mood diary can be kept for a set period of time (Table 12.2). This records all food and beverage intake, time of intake and requires the person to rate their mood at that time.

Exercise

- What amount of exercise does he do in a day?
- Is he interested in any team sports?
- Is he interested in individual sport?
- How long is it since he regularly participated in any sporting activities?
- Has he put on any weight?
- If so, why does he think he has put on weight?
- Over what period of time has he noticed his weight gain?
- What would he like to do about it?
- Is he interested in participating in an exercise programme?

Table 12.2 Food/mood diary.

Day ....   Date ....   Weight ....

Meal	Time	Food eaten	Quantity	Where eaten	Mood/events	Water
Breakfast						
Morn. tea						
Lunch						
Aft. tea						
Dinner						
Supper						
Additional						

To assess various physical activities, you could use the Health and Nutrition Examination Survey (National Center for Health Statistics, 1973). You could use a simple survey like the one below to give you some idea about Sam's level of activity and what he is interested in. This survey has been adapted from the Active Australia Survey (Australian Institute of Health and Welfare, 2003). It is available on the internet and is free of charge.

The following questions are to find out about the different types of physical activity you did over the past week.

1. In the past week, how many times have you walked for recreation or exercise and/or to do errands for at least 10 minutes continuously? _____times
    Please estimate the total time you spent walking in the past week.
    _____hours/_____minutes
2. In the past week, how many times did you do vigorous exercise or other physical activity (in your leisure time or at work) which made you breather harder or puff or pant (e.g. jogging or running, heavy gardening, netball, chopping wood, vigorous swimming, heavy labouring, etc.)? _____times
    Please estimate the total time you spent doing vigorous exercise or physical activity in the past week.
    _____hours/_____minutes
3. In the past week, how many times did you do moderate exercise or other physical activity (in your leisure time or at work) which did not make you breather harder or puff and pant (e.g. more moderate activities such as digging in the garden, moderate cycling, raking leaves, dancing, etc.)? _____times
    Please estimate the total time you spent doing moderate exercise or physical activity in the past week.
    _____hours/_____minutes
4. In the past week, was there any time when you thought about exercising but didn't? What stopped you?
5. The next question is about your leisure time – that time when you are not working, travelling to work or sleeping (Table 12.3).

Table 12.3   How do you spend your leisure time?

Activity	Total hours/ minutes Monday to Friday	Total hours/ minutes Saturday and Sunday
Hobbies, e.g. arts/crafts, work on car, play musical instrument		
Reading, e.g. books, papers, magazines		
Sitting and socialising, e.g. with friends and family (at home, pubs, restaurants, etc.)		
Sitting or lying and listening to music/radio		
Talking on the telephone		
Watching TV/DVDs (including video games)		
Using the computer (including the internet, games)		
Going for drive		
Relaxing, thinking, resting (not including sleeping)		
Other inactive recreation (specify)		

Step 2: Deciding on a program for Sam

You will need to decide whether Sam would be best off attending a group programme in rehabilitation or whether some individual sessions would be more effective. This decision is usually based on the person's circumstances. In this particular case, Sam has been feeling bored and is sitting around not doing much with his time. After discussion with Sam, you both decide that a group programme would suit him best as this would give him a chance to start interacting with other people who are similar to him. You refer him to two group programmes, one a substance misuse program and the other a healthy lifestyle programme.

The substance misuse group programme is designed for young adults under 30 years, as their issues and needs may be different from those of older adults who may have had substance use issues for a longer period of time. Between six and eight clients are included to enable a sense of group cohesion and trust to develop. This particular group programme is run during business hours over an 8-week period and each session is 3 hours in duration. The preferred venue for this group is a neutral community setting which is considered to be less stigmatising.

As well as information giving and sharing, clients engage in goal setting, discussions, brainstorming, role play and practical experiences. Handouts are used to reinforce content. Active participation in leisure activities provides clients with practical experiences that enhance their wellbeing and enables them to experience alternative ways of obtaining satisfaction and enjoyment. This programme may be modified if you need to conduct individual sessions with the client.

A substance misuse group programme

Session 1: Introduction

The introductory group is facilitated by the group leader(s). In this session, the facilitators introduce themselves to the group members and discuss the outline of the programme.

Discuss concepts of interactive style of education and participation in positive substance-free fun/leisure activities weekly. Have the participants introduce themselves to the group. Ask what stops people from participating in leisure activities and how their substance use affects their participation.

Explore group participants' expectations

List participants' goals and expectations from attending the group.

Getting acquainted

Use warm-up activities to enable participants to get to know each other and to explore their strengths and areas they want to work on.

The recovery journey

Identify where participants are in the journey by providing them with a diagram of a road where one end represents the achievement of their desired goal and the other represents the beginning of the journey. Ask participants to indicate where they are on the road and encourage them to explore where they are in relation to others in the group.

Stages of Change Model

Explain that change may occur when the costs versus benefits of behaviours are considered. Explore the pros and cons of substance use with participants. Identify discrepancies between the pros and cons to understand the participants' decisional balance. Discuss the Stages of Change Model and determine the stage participants are at.

Baseline assessment

Use standardised measures.

Session evaluation

Ask participants to circle words that describe how they felt about the session, things they enjoyed the most, things they would like to change and one thing they will take away from the session.

Leisure activity

Participate in an activity selected by the group, for example bush walking.

Session 2: Coping with cravings

The introduction and warm-up exercise are facilitated by the group leader.

Effects of intoxication

This is an information-giving section facilitated by the group leader. This addresses the effects of intoxication and withdrawal and the influence of substance use on mental health.

Awareness of cravings

Ask the group members to describe their cravings, if they have them. Brainstorm and discuss ideas about delaying cravings. Emphasise the importance of distraction and engaging in activities not connected with using.

Changing negative self-talk

Discuss how negative self-talk and beliefs can often lead to lapsing into substance use. Provide a handout on steps to changing thinking, challenging negative thinking, demanding evidence, reasoning it out, substituting with a better option, replacing the word 'should' with 'could', giving oneself permission to feel good. Ask participants to tell the group one positive thing about themselves or their progress.

Session evaluation

The evaluation of the session is the same as for session 1.

Leisure activity

Participate in an activity selected by the group, for example swimming.

Session 3: Communication

The introduction and warm-up exercise are facilitated by the group leader.

Communication

Brainstorm ideas about effective communication. Discuss how people's perceptions of an event can be masked by their substance use. Discuss communication differences when using and not using substances.

Problem solving

What is a problem? How do problems affect participants? How do they currently solve problems? Discuss problems experienced by group participants and possible solutions. Provide a handout on steps to solve problems – identify thoughts and feelings about the problems, define the problem, identify alternatives, choose an option, create an action plan and practise. Role play an exercise in problem solving.

Session evaluation

Complete the session evaluation as for session 1.

Leisure activity

Participate in an activity selected by the group, for example volleyball.

Session 4: Planning for high-risk situations

The introduction and warm-up exercise are facilitated by the group leader.

What to do in high-risk situations

Brainstorm ideas.

Skills to cope with relapse triggers

Discuss signs and signals of stress reactions and coping skills. Ask group participants to identify stressful situations. Discuss how these situations can be reframed. Discuss positive affirmations. Practise relaxation techniques.

Session evaluation

This is the same as for session 1.

Leisure activity

Participate in an activity selected by the group, for example canoeing.

Session 5: Setting goals

The introduction and warm-up exercise are facilitated by the group leader.

Goal setting

Information giving facilitated by the group leader. Brainstorm what goals are and how to set them. Provide a handout on principles of goal setting, making goals observable, realistic, achievable and action oriented. Look at the steps involved in successful goal setting. Practise setting a goal. Ask the group to say one positive thing that they have achieved since the group started.

Time use

Discuss time use. Complete a time pie. Discuss good time management.

Session evaluation

This is the same as for session 1.

Leisure activity

Participate in an activity selected by the group, for example basketball.

Session 6: Substance refusal skills

The introduction and warm-up exercise are facilitated by the group leader.

Drink refusal skills

Information giving by the group leader. Ask participants to describe situations in which they had problems refusing substances. Brainstorm more assertive responses. Role play refusal of substances. Discuss what it was like for participants in the role play and for those watching. Provide a handout on drink refusal skills, for example verbal strategies ('not for me, thanks'), non-verbal strategies (using body language and eye contact), alternatives (change the subject, request that the other person stop asking them to use).

Conflict resolution, assertiveness and anger management

Information giving by group leader about verbal and non-verbal behaviour, assertive behaviour and anger. Brainstorm personal experiences of anger. Provide a handout on anger management solutions, for example taking time out, changing the focus, addressing one's thinking (don't personalise or jump to conclusions), and go through it with the group. Look at what is assertive behaviour. Role play an alternative way of expressing anger using recent scenarios provided by a participant. General discussion about how they felt about the activity.

Session evaluation

This is the same as for session 1.

Leisure activity

Participate in an activity selected by the group, for example ten-pin bowling.

Session 7: Lifestyle changes

Introduction and warm-up activity are facilitated by the group leader.

Finding alternatives to substance use

Identify interests and current activity levels. What are the participants interested in? List participants' desired lifestyle changes. Identify barriers to making changes and discuss barriers to making changes. Explore ways to overcome barriers.

Community resources and services

Provide a handout on resources and services in the local area. Get group members to identify one positive aspect of joining community groups by the end of the session.

Changing negative self-talk

Discuss negative self-talk and the importance of positive affirmations.

Session evaluation

This is the same as for session 1.

Leisure activity

Participate in an activity selected by the group, for example tennis.

Session 8: Leisure

Introduction and warm-up activity are facilitated by the group leader.

Importance of leisure

Discuss the benefits of leisure participation and planning for the future. Discuss the importance of keeping active.

Leisure activity

Participate in an activity selected by the group, for example a BBQ.

Readminister baseline assessment and complete overall evaluation of the group. It may be useful to evaluate the leisure component of the programme with the Leisure Motivation Scale (Beard & Ragheb, 1983).

Celebrate completion of the group programme. Hand out certificates of attendance.

Healthy lifestyle programme

In addition to the substance misuse programme, you decide that a lifestyle group would be beneficial for Sam. Lifestyle groups are useful for any clients for whom poor lifestyle habits have been identified. Clients with psychotic disorders comprise the majority of clients in these programmes because poor nutritional intake and physical inactivity are significant issues for them (Catapano & Castle, 2003; McLeod *et al.*, 2009).

This particular lifestyle group is run over 9 weeks, with 2-hourly sessions twice weekly. Clients are given the opportunity to continue in the group for the following 9 weeks to consolidate their skills and lifestyle changes.

This programme requires a venue with a sizeable group room and ready access to cooking facilities for the nutritional component. If these facilities are not available, individual work may be more effective. Other practical components take place at a local supermarket and gym. It is important that Sam is checked out by the GP to make sure he doesn't have any physical problems that would be compounded by attending the fitness programme.

This group programme assists clients to set goals with regard to their nutritional intake, spending habits and physical activity levels. In the nutritional and budgeting sections of the group programme, the principal approach involves the use of a proportional spending model, which means demonstrating that the nutritional quality of a person's diet can be improved by changing the proportion of funds available to spend on various types of foods. Clients are assisted to balance their diet and food budget and to understand how good nutrition and physical activity work together to achieve a healthy lifestyle.

Fitness

The fitness component of the group programme consists of a 15-minute warm-up, a 30-minute circuit or exercise class and a cooldown session. Clients are also involved in developing an activity plan and setting goals. So even though people do exercises in the programme, there is a need to emphasise that exercise needs to be incorporated into everyday activity. It may be useful to talk to Sam about getting involved in some of the programmes sponsored by local authorities. You could help Sam search the web for free or low-cost programmes offered by city councils or other organisations. He can also locate his nearest park or other places where he would be able to engage in healthy activities. Sam might also consider trying out an activity he has never done before by joining a beginner's group. Many activities are offered at minimal cost and some are free. The sessions offered by the council cater to all ages and fitness levels.

Explain that physical activity is something that everyone can enjoy and point out that making activity a regular part of your day has lots of benefits to health and wellbeing.

Box 12.1 lists of some of the activities that might be available.

Box 12.1   Possible physical activities

Cycling – this may be through the wetlands, along the river, down to the beach, etc.
Surfing
Kayaking
Fishing
Visiting the botanical gardens
Tai chi
Belly dancing
Meditation
Running group
Triathlon
Tennis
Softball
Bushcare (rivers, parks, wetlands, beaches)
Community gardens
Paddleboarding

Skating
Boxing for fitness
Walking group
Pilates
Yoga
Aqua aerobics
Swimming
Bowls
Line dancing
Kung fu and Chinese Wushu
Frisbees
Nature lovers – bees, frogs, birdwatching, nocturnal animals
Skiing
Windsurfing
Skateboarding

Box 12.2   How to make physical activity more enjoyable

Make physical activity a part of your regular routine	Start slowly and progress gradually. Start with a 10-minute walk and gradually increase the time
Walk wherever you can	Make sure you balance physical activity with healthy eating for the best results
Use the stairs instead of escalators, elevators or lifts	Buy a pedometer so that you can count your steps. Aim for 10,000 steps a day

---

It may also be useful to give Sam some tips to help him find the time and make physical activity fun and more enjoyable. Some tips are listed in Box 12.2.

The fitness component of the lifestyle programme is addressed below.

- Let's get fit – strategies.
- Goal setting – what participants want to achieve.
- Physical activity plan – what activity, when, how many minutes.
- Addressing lifestyle changes.
- Initial weigh-in.
- Exercise: 15-minute warm-up, 30-minute circuit/exercise class, cooldown. This exercise schedule is repeated on a weekly basis for the duration of the group.
- Stress importance of physical activity for the body – for example, improves metabolism, bone strength, cardiovascular circulation, mental state and concentration.
- Stress types of physical activity and their benefits – for example, aerobic, weight bearing, moderate intensity and vigorous intensity.
- Give beneficial physical activity levels, for example, moderate-intensity activity totalling a minimum of 30 minutes/day most days/week (this is repeated from the first component of the programme).
- Three-weekly evaluation –weight and body fat percentage levels.
- Computer printout of all measurements since commencement of group.
- Attend the graduation group of the lifestyle programme.

Healthy eating

To run the following healthy eating sessions, the group leaders will need to prepare the activities and make sure all food ingredients and food preparation utensils are readily available.

Session 1: Food for life – strategies

- Introduction and warm-up exercise.
- Establish understanding of food groups/nutrition.
- Introduction to the food pyramid which classifies food according to how much should be eaten to achieve optimal nutrition (Nutrition Australia 2003).
- Activity requiring the group to classify food pictures and/or packets according to the food pyramid.

- Introduce food preparation skills. Activities could include the washing of fruit and vegetables; how to chop fruit and vegetables; basic food hygiene around use of chopping boards; and basic safety on knife handling.

Session 2: Eating for life

- Revise five food groups.
- Reinforce concepts of the healthy diet pyramid.
- Identify where individual foods fit into the pyramid.
- Look at a simple food recipe such as cheese on toast. Group members identify the food groups involved and how often this kind of food should be eaten.
- Continue food preparation skills including safe use of electrical appliances in kitchen; safe use of grater.

Session 3: Life is for living

- Revise five food groups.
- Reinforce concepts of the healthy diet pyramid.
- Discuss quantities of different foods in a balanced diet. Look at healthy portion sizes and compare to portion sizes group members normally use.
- Prepare a corned beef and salad sandwich, scrambled eggs or a tuna salad.
- Continue food preparation skills including safe use of electrical appliances; safe use of hotplate; washing-up techniques.

Session 4: Balanced for life

- Stress importance of physical activity for the body – for example, improves metabolism, bone strength, cardiovascular circulation, mental state and concentration.
- Give beneficial physical activity levels, for example, moderate-intensity activity totalling a minimum of 30 minutes/day most days/week.
- Find out what types of physical activity each person is doing in their free time.
- Discuss what constitutes a healthy snack. Prepare a fruit and nut platter. Discuss healthy portion sizes.
- Continue food preparation skills: safe use of knives; washing of fruit; use of chopping boards; washing-up skills.

Session 5: Planning for life – Food Cent$, Part 1 (Foley, 1998)

- Plan a healthy meal for breakfast, lunch and dinner.
- Review healthy diet pyramid, noting where the food for each meal fits and then discuss the overall healthy status of the meal.
- Introduce the 10-plan by using the healthy diet pyramid as a guide – that is, one part in the 'eat least' foods, three parts in the 'eat moderately' foods and six parts in the 'eat most' foods. Compare how the meals selected fit with the 10-plan.

- Prepare the lunch meal.
- Continue food preparation skills, e.g. food hygiene; safe use of kitchen appliances; safe use of knives; washing-up techniques; introduce safe food storage, focusing on refrigeration and freezing of food.
- For the next week, encourage clients to bring in their grocery bills for the session.

Session 6: Planning for life –Food Cent$, Part 2

- Discuss the 10-plan and how it fits into the client's food budget, i.e. divide food budget by 10 and allocate money to each food group of the pyramid proportionally.
- Allocate grocery budget according to nutritional value of foods, that is, spending most on the 'eat most' foods.
- Ask members to examine their own shopping habits (use client grocery bills) and apply the 10-plan shopping routine.
- Prepare pumpkin soup for lunch. While preparing, review how soup fits into the healthy diet pyramid and then how cost would fit to the 10-plan. In light of these, discuss if this is a healthy meal.
- Continue food preparation skills including blending; use of knives; use of appliances; food hygiene; safety in the kitchen; food storage.

Session 7: Shopping for life – Food Cent$, Part 3

- Revise the 10-plan budgeting guide and use the Kilo Cent$ counter (see below) in the practical context of the supermarket.
- Discuss that more processed 'convenience' foods are usually more expensive.
- Compare the cost of different foods using the price per kilogram.
- Use the Kilo Cent$ counter to find and compare the cost per kilogram of different foods.
- Identify cheaper, more nutritious alternatives to processed foods.
- Discuss the need to carefully consider food costs and nutritional value when shopping.
- Buy ingredients for a picnic from the supermarket using the 10-plan.
- Have a picnic in a nearby park.

The Kilo Cent$ counter was designed by Western Australian dieticians as a means of comparing food prices. It is a table that has the weights down one side and the prices along the top (Figure 12.1). To use the tool, you look for the weight of the food item and then the price. You move along the corresponding column and row until they meet. The value listed where they meet is the cost of 1 kilogram of that food item. By using this tool, people are able to compare the cost of food types by comparing the cost for 1 kilogram for both food types. An example of this would be a kilogram of fresh apples compared to a kilo of pie apples. By using the Kilo Cent$ counter, you would be able to work out which was more expensive. The Kilo Cent$ counter could easily be converted to use the currency of any country. In some countries, such as Australia, supermarkets are now required by law to include the cost per 100 g on the

The Kilo Cent$ counter

Grams	50c	$1.00	$1.50	$2.00	$2.50	$3.00	$3.50	$4.00	$4.50	$5.00
50	10.00	20.00	30.00	40.00	50.00	60.00	70.00	80.00	90.00	100.00
100	5.00	10.00	15.00	20.00	25.00	30.00	35.00	40.00	45.00	50.00
150	3.33	6.67	10.00	13.33	16.67	20.00	23.33	26.67	30.00	33.33
200	2.50	5.00	7.50	10.00	12.50	15.00	17.50	20.00	22.50	25.00
250	2.00	4.00	6.00	8.00	10.00	12.00	14.00	16.00	18.00	20.00
300	1.67	3.33	5.00	6.67	8.33	10.00	11.67	13.33	15.00	16.67
350	1.43	2.86	4.28	5.71	7.14	8.57	10.00	11.43	12.86	14.28
400	1.25	2.50	3.75	5.00	6.25	7.50	8.75	10.00	11.25	12.50
450	1.11	2.22	3.33	4.44	5.56	6.67	7.78	8.89	10.00	11.11
500	1.00	2.00	3.00	4.00	5.00	6.00	7.00	8.00	9.00	10.00
550	0.91	1.82	2.73	3.64	4.54	5.45	6.36	7.27	8.18	9.09
600	0.83	1.67	2.50	3.33	4.17	5.00	5.83	6.67	7.50	8.33
650	0.77	1.54	2.31	3.08	3.85	4.61	5.38	6.15	6.92	7.69
700	0.71	1.43	2.14	2.86	3.57	4.28	5.00	5.71	6.43	7.14
750	0.67	1.33	2.00	2.67	3.33	4.00	4.67	5.33	6.00	6.67
800	0.62	1.25	1.87	2.50	3.12	3.75	4.37	5.00	5.62	6.25
850	0.59	1.18	1.76	2.35	2.94	3.53	4.12	4.70	5.29	5.88
900	0.55	1.10	1.67	2.22	2.78	3.33	3.89	4.44	5.00	5.56
950	0.53	1.05	1.58	2.10	2.63	3.16	3.68	4.21	4.74	5.26
1000	0.50	1.00	1.50	2.00	2.50	3.00	3.50	4.00	4.50	5.00

Price

ML	$5.50	$6.00	$6.50	$7.00	$7.50	$8.00	$8.50	$9.00	$9.50	$10.00
50	110.00	120.00	130.00	140.00	150.00	160.00	170.00	180.00	190.00	200.00
100	55.00	60.00	65.00	70.00	75.00	80.00	85.00	90.00	95.00	100.00
150	36.67	40.00	43.33	46.66	50.00	53.33	56.67	60.00	63.33	66.66
200	27.50	30.00	32.50	35.00	37.50	40.00	42.50	45.00	47.50	50.00
250	22.00	24.00	26.00	28.00	30.00	32.00	34.00	36.00	38.00	40.00
300	18.33	20.00	21.67	23.34	25.00	26.66	28.33	30.00	31.67	33.34
350	15.71	17.14	18.57	20.00	21.43	22.86	24.29	25.72	27.14	28.56
400	13.75	15.00	16.25	17.50	18.75	20.00	21.25	22.50	33.75	25.00
450	12.23	13.34	14.45	15.56	16.67	17.78	18.89	20.00	21.11	22.22
500	11.00	12.00	13.00	14.00	15.00	16.00	17.00	18.00	19.00	20.00
550	10.00	10.90	11.81	12.72	13.63	14.54	15.35	16.36	17.27	18.18
600	9.17	10.00	10.83	11.66	12.50	13.34	14.17	15.00	15.83	16.66
650	8.46	9.22	10.00	10.76	11.53	12.30	13.07	13.84	14.61	15.38
700	7.85	8.56	9.28	10.00	10.71	11.42	12.14	12.86	13.57	14.28
750	7.33	8.00	8.67	9.34	10.00	10.66	11.33	12.00	12.67	13.34
800	6.87	7.50	8.12	8.74	9.37	10.00	10.62	11.24	11.87	12.50
850	6.47	7.06	7.65	8.24	8.82	9.40	10.00	10.58	11.17	11.76
900	6.11	6.66	7.22	7.78	8.33	8.88	9.44	10.00	10.56	11.12
950	5.79	6.32	6.84	7.36	7.89	8.42	8.95	9.47	10.00	10.52
1000	5.50	6.00	6.50	7.00	7.50	8.00	8.50	9.00	9.50	10.00

Price

1000 g = 1 kg

1000 ml = 1 litre

Figure 12.1 The Kilo Cent$ counter.

shelf price tag. This effectively does the same thing as the Kilo Cent$ counter. It allows for the comparison of prices for food items.

Session 8: Food for life

* Review budgeting, healthy eating and value for money concepts discussed over the past weeks as part of the Food Cent$ component.
* Discus information obtained from the practical activity in the last session.
* Identify foods that were good value for money and those that were not.
* Discuss the differences between the cost of convenience food and standard food items.
* Identify changes to personal shopping habits.
* Decide on a menu for graduation the following week including entrée, main and dessert using the healthy food pyramid and the 10-plan.
* Clients are encouraged to invite one guest to the graduation session next week. Guests are to arrive for the last hour of the session.
* Prepare an egg dish for lunch.
* Continue food preparation skills including whisking food; safety in the kitchen; food hygiene; food storage; safe use of electrical appliances; safe use of knives and other kitchen utensils.

Graduation

* Shop for food.
* Prepare food according to menu drawn up last week. Could be done by small work groups, e.g. one group doing the soup, etc.
* Have the meal.
* Clean up.
* Presentation of graduation certificates.

Home visits

It may be useful to include a number of home visits to check how Sam is actually doing with the program (Table 12.4). Home visits are very helpful to ensure that learning in the programme can be transferred into daily life. When undertaking home visits, it is important to observe safety protocols. These may include ensuring you are accompanied (especially when visiting people who are not well known to you), ensuring colleagues know where you are, carrying a mobile phone with speed dial and arranging for family members to be present.

We suggest that you commence with a baseline observation of Sam and then visit him every 3 weeks of the programme. Perhaps it might be useful to visit him again 3 weeks after the conclusion of the programme to see if he has adopted any of the information provided to him in the group programme. It is probably a good idea to phone Sam first and ask him if he is able to prepare a simple snack for lunch while you visit.

Table 12.4 Home visit schedule.

Frequency	Activities
Baseline	Phone and arrange to visit Sam. Introduce yourself and tell Sam about the healthy lifestyle programme. Ask Sam the questions listed under diet. Identify cooking resources and equipment and discuss these with Sam to determine his knowledge and familiarity concerning their use. Explore ways of acquiring essential items that are missing. Observe Sam preparing a snack for lunch. Observe Sam's food preparation skills. Check his food storage areas including the refrigerator
Three-weekly	Check with Sam his understanding of the healthy diet pyramid. Check Sam's groceries and his understanding of where these foods fit into the pyramid. Observe him preparing something he learned about in the group
Six-weekly	Check with Sam about his level of physical activity. Discuss with Sam about what he understands to be a healthy snack. Discuss with Sam the 10-plan and how the food he has fits into the 10-plan. Ask Sam what he plans to prepare for his evening meal and review availability of necessary ingredients, utensils and equipment. Look at Sam's food budget for the week and how he allocates money to each food group
Nine-weekly	Review budgeting, healthy eating and value for money. Discuss the need to carefully consider food costs. Explore how he found the programme and what specifically has changed about his diet and exercise
Follow-up (3 weeks after end of programme)	Review with Sam about how he is doing, is he using the 10-plan budgeting guide, has he noticed any changes to the amount of money he is spending per week on groceries, has he changed his personal shopping habits? Discuss fitness and exercise habits and review weight and plans for maintaining any gains

Summary

You met with Sam and administered some basic screening instruments to assess his food intake, his activity levels and his readiness to change. After discussion, you and Sam both agreed that attending a group programme would be most beneficial for him. The programmes that Sam attended were the substance misuse programme and the healthy living programme. To assess Sam's progress, you conducted regular home visits at 3-week intervals. You and Sam decided that it would be helpful for him if he attended the group programme and learnt a bit more about budgeting and transportation so Sam enrolled in the subsequent rehabilitation group programme to address these issues. Lifestyle programmes are particularly important for people with mental illness. Compared to the general population, individuals with schizophrenia display increased rates of obesity and have a higher risk of premature death from heart disease and cerebrovascular accidents. Potential causes include poor diet and physical inactivity (McLeod et al., 2009). A single programme such as we have described may be very helpful in getting a person started on lifestyle change but maintaining changes is a lifelong project.

References

Australian Institute of Health and Welfare (2003) *The Active Australia Survey: A Guide and Manual for Implementation, Analysis, and Reporting.* Australian Institute of Health and Welfare: Canberra.

Beard J, Ragheb M (1983) Measuring leisure motivation. *Journal of Leisure Research* **15**, 219–28.

Catapano L, Castle D (2003) Obesity in schizophrenia: what can be done about it? *Australasian Psychiatry* **12**, 23–5.

Foley R (1998) The Food Cent$ project: a practical application of behaviour change theory. *Australian Journal of Nutrition and Dietetics* **55**, 33–5.

McLeod HJ, Jacques S, Deane FP (2009) Base rates of physical activity in Australians with schizophrenia. *Psychiatric Rehabilitation Journal* **32**, 261–7.

National Center for Health Statistics (1973) *Plan and Operation of the Health and Nutrition Examination Survey, United States 1971–1973*. National Center for Health Statistics: Rockville, MD.

Nutrition Australia (2003) www.nutritionaustralia.com

Raistrick D, Dunbar G, Davidson R (1983) Development of a questionnaire to measure alcohol dependence. *British Journal of Addiction* **78**, 89–95.

Rollnick S, Healther N, Gold R, Hall W (1992) Development of a short 'readiness to change' questionnaire for use in brief, opportunistic interventions among excessive drinkers. *British Journal of Addictions* **87**, 743–54.

Sanders J, Aasland O, Babor T, de la Fuente J, Grant M (1993) Development of the Alcohol Use Disorders Identification Test (AUDIT). WHO collaborative project on early detection of persons with harmful alcohol consumption – II. *Addiction* **88**, 791–804. A copy of the Alcohol Use Disorders Identification Test (AUDIT) and manual is available free of charge from www.who.int/substance_abuse/docs/audit2.pdf.

Chapter 13

Living Skills

Chris Lloyd and Hazel Bassett

> After the completion of the previous programme and in the follow-up home visit, Sam identifies that he still has problems with cooking and wishes to do something about that. He also identifies that he has problems with his budget and isn't able to prioritise his spending. Further discussion reveals that Sam has problems with transportation. While he is able to get around if he can drive, he does not currently have a car of his own and has been relying on Angela to take him places he could easily get to using public transport. The fact is that he has no idea how to use public transport.

After your home visits with Sam, observation of how he was managing and further discussion, you and Sam agree on a number of areas that he would benefit from learning more about. These include:

• money management
• transportation
• cooking.

Sam has agreed to re-engage with rehabilitation to address these specific issues. Although this information could be presented individually, you decide that a group programme would be more appropriate for Sam. You base this decision on Sam's current situation. Factors you consider include:

• isolation
• lack of friends and connection
• difficulty with basic living skills.

You decide that Sam would be better off attending a group programme where he could mix with other young people who are experiencing similar problems. Attending a group programme will provide Sam with the opportunity to make friends and to learn from other people about some of the issues that they have experienced and some of the possible solutions they have found.

Manual of Psychosocial Rehabilitation, First Edition. Edited by Robert King, Chris Lloyd, Tom Meehan, Frank P. Deane and David J. Kavanagh.
© 2012 Blackwell Publishing Ltd. Published 2012 by Blackwell Publishing Ltd.

Money managing/budgeting group

A group that focuses on money management/budgeting can teach people skills in the areas of:

- identifying priorities for money usage such as buying food, medication, paying rent, having money for leisure activities, etc.
- identifying their own spending habits
- setting goals for how they will spend their money
- developing a budget
- exploring savings plans.

It is hoped that through the group, the group members would develop their own budget. Another outcome would be the sharing of ideas about how to budget and any strategies that they have identified that have helped in the past. Often it is not the knowledge of the practitioner but the sharing of ideas by group members that assists people in developing and trying new strategies. A secondary outcome of the group is the interaction of group members and the friendships that may develop.

The programme could be delivered on an individual basis but the sharing and developing of friendships would not then occur.

Session 1: Introducing the group

- What the group is about.
- Warm-up activity (for examples of warm-up activities, see Chapter 11 and Box 13.1).
- Identifying priorities and values.
- Lead discussion around what activities constitutes self-improvement, family life, special interests, study and leisure.
- Use of a worksheet where participants are asked to rate the following, with 1 being their greatest priority: self-improvement, family life, special interests, study and leisure.
- Group discussion: exploring priorities and relevance of these to individual or family wants and needs. Also discuss how they make decisions around the expenditure of their money.
- Do they consider that they have problems concerning the items purchased?
- Is this something they would like to work on?
- Ask group members to identify any problem areas.
- Cooldown activity (for examples of cooldown activities, see Chapter 11 and Box 13.2).
- Homework activity: keep a diary of all expenditures for the week and rate their priority.

Session 2: Awareness of spending habits

- Warm-up activity.
- Use a worksheet which outlines spending habits.
- After completion of the worksheet, there is a group discussion about participants' spending style, e.g. considered, spur of the moment, easily talked into, ask others, etc.

Box 13.1   Warm-up exercises

Exercise 1 – Tissue exercise	Group members to pretend they have a cold. Group members to pull out enough tissues to use for one day with a cold. Then taking turns, members share one thing about self for each tissue taken, e.g. favourite colour, food, animal, music, interests, etc.
Exercise 2 – My horoscope	Tell group you are drawing an imaginary line down the middle of the room with January at one end of the room and December the other. Ask the group to line up on the line in order of month and date of birth. Group members to read out their own horoscope to the group.
Exercise 3 – A famous person	Taking turns, ask group members to identify a famous person, e.g. film star, author, singer, etc. that they admire and give reasons why they admire that person.
Exercise 4 – Find the change	Ask group for a volunteer. Ask that person to go outside and change something about their appearance, e.g. undo more buttons, turn hat around, etc. When the person returns, the group is to identify the changes. If time allows, repeat exercise.
Exercise 5 – Auction	Items to be auctioned are placed in the middle of the group. Member volunteers to be the auctioneer and choose the item and auction it off to the group.
Exercise 6 – Mirrors	Members to find themselves a partner, whom they feel at ease with. Members to face each other and make eye contact and try and maintain it throughout. One member moves a part or parts of body very slowly, while the other tries to mirror the motion. The pair then switches roles. Provide an opportunity for group to discuss any feelings they may have experienced.
Exercise 7 – Feelings	Hand out a sheet of paper to all group members. Ask them to draw how they are feeling today. Discuss as a group.
Exercise 8 – Rhythm cycle	Explain to the group that they will be making music using noises they can make using their bodies. One member starts off making a sound, then going around the circle, the group joins in one at a time, until all members are making music. After a short time, members stop making their own music one by one, with the person who started the music finishing first.
Exercise 9 – Chinese whisper	Members sit in a circle. One member is asked to think of a sentence or phrase and whisper it in the ear of the person sitting next to them. This continues until the last person repeats out loud the message heard and compares it to the original message.
Exercise 10 – Non-verbal communication	Group to form into pairs. Ask members to have a conversation using drawing with coloured crayons. Pairs to share one piece of paper.

- Evaluation of participants' spending style by reviewing the homework activity and have people consider why they spent what they did.
- Discussion as to whether there are issues they are willing to address.
- Identify ideas for making changes in this area and share with the group.
- Cooldown activity.
- Homework: continue to keep diary of spending. Note transaction details, e.g. cash, credit, direct debit, bill paying, etc. Note spending style for each transaction. Also consider priority of item purchased.

Box 13.2   Cooldown activities

Activity 1   Taking turns, group members are asked to identify one thing they like/admire about another group member's appearance.

Activity 2   Explain to members that you will be calling out certain personal traits, e.g. find someone with the same coloured eyes as you have, find someone with the same coloured hair as you have. Members are to find and stand with a person with whom they share these characteristics.

Activity 3   Write the word 'friend' on the board and ask group members to identify different words they can make out of this word.

Activity 4   Group members are given a sheet of paper. They write their name on the sheet and then pass their sheet to the person next to them. This person writes a compliment about the person whose name is on the sheet. This continues until all group members have a written compliment on all sheets. Taking turns, group members then read out the compliments written on their sheet.

Activity 5   Group members to share an experience with the group that they once felt embarrassed about, but have learnt from that experience and can look back and laugh.

Activity 6   Hand out a sheet of paper and pens to each person. Ask members to tear the sheet of paper so that they have the same number of pieces as there are people in the group. Participants write the names of fellow group members on each piece of paper and then a gift or wish they would like to give that person. When everybody is finished, ask members to give their slips of paper to the appropriate person. Each person is then invited to read out their collection of gifts.

Session 3: Setting goals

- Warm-up activity.
- Discussion centring on what goals serve as a guide to spending.
- Have a collection of catalogues containing items for purchase such as furniture, food, clothing, music and entertainment, travel, etc. (junk mail would be useful). Ask participants to look at the catelogues and then write down all the things they would like that money can buy.
- Ask them to identify which of these are important for the person now and what is important for the future.
- Discussion: consider homework and have participants identify how important each of the items is to them. Have participants think about what their goals are with regard to their spending. Invite participants to share two of their short-term goals.
- Ask participants to identify if these are realistic in terms of their income and expenses.
- Check with them about whether they think their family would agree with them.
- Ask participants to discuss how they might reach some of these goals.
- Cooldown activity.
- Homework: collect up last month's bills and bring them in for the next session.

Session 4: Identifying monthly expenses

- Warm-up activity.
- Give participants a worksheet for them to list their expenses and the approximate amount they spend. Have the participants also include the bills they have brought in for homework.
- Discussion: do participants live within their income, what are their problem areas, which expenses do they think they can cut down on, are they able to meet any short- or long-term goals with their present spending pattern, how can this be changed?
- Explore some of the cheaper options for shopping, e.g. charity shop for clothing, home-band food items.
- Cooldown activity.
- Homework: participants source cheaper options for themselves in all areas listed in session 1, e.g. walk instead of catching the bus if they don't have far to go.

Session 5: Making a budget

- Warm-up activity.
- Discuss that an important aspect of setting up a budget is identifying which expenses are fixed and which are flexible.
- Ask participants to identify what their fixed expenses are.
- Then get them to identify their flexible expenses. Ask the group to assist with ideas about how these can be cut down. Consider some of the options they have come up with in the homework activity.
- Discuss the issue of the next time you feel the urge to buy and ways to counter this. Ask questions such as:
  - Will I be pleased with my purchases?
  - Am I able to afford this?
  - Do I want to spend my money on this right now?
  - Why am I really buying this?
  - Am I OK with my reasons for making this purchase?
- Cooldown activity.
- Homework: work up an individual budget considering all fixed expenses and changing expenses. Consider a realistic saving goal for each week and identify a goal to save for.

Session 6: Resources and requirements

- Warm-up activity.
- Discussion centring around the resources of clients, i.e. time, money, energy, ability, knowledge, equipment.
- Discussion then focuses on knowing individual requirements, i.e. how will it be used, how long will it last, what features are the most important, what quality is necessary? Review homework and have each participant share the goal that they will attempt to save for.
- Cooldown activity.

Conclusion

Although the programme outlined here is designed for a group, it is possible to use much of the content and resources to conduct the session individually with Sam. If your client lives with their parents, you could also include them in the sessions. It is most important that the person is encouraged to do the homework sessions as this will give the facilitator a good idea of how the client is progressing and will also provide some additional information to work with in the subsequent session.

Transportation

Sam has difficulty getting to his rehabilitation programme and with attending appointments. As the area is well serviced by trains, trams, buses and ferries, you and Sam discuss where he needs to go and what would be the best form of transportation to get him to those places. It appears that the bus would be suitable for the things that Sam needs to do. Depending on what transportation is required, the programme would focus on that. This particular programme is conducted individually although it could be conducted in a group format. The number of sessions is flexible and depends on the client's level of skill and confidence in being able to access public transport. It will be necessary for the facilitator to have good knowledge about where transport information can be found. For example, this would include the local bus depot, information provided at major bus stops, information provided via the telephone or local transportation websites.

A programme devoted to exploring public transport options focuses on developing skills in the areas of:

- exploring timetables, maps and the use of the internet to find information
- planning and scheduling activities and transport.

The objective of the programme is to build skills that will assist the person to plan an outing and then use public transport to get there.

Session 1: Introducing the programme

- Getting baseline information from the participant and determining the most suitable form of transport to use.
- Has he ever used public transport? Or is it a skill that has become rusty with disuse? Is he uncomfortable in the presence of strangers?
- What does the participant need to access?
- How many times per week?
- Does he think he can budget for this?
- Check what he would like to achieve by the end of the programme (goals).

Session 2: Bus timetables and maps

You may need to repeat this session a number of times for the person to feel comfortable accessing transport. It is best to focus it around places that the person needs to go and at similar times to when he will be going.

- Review public transport maps.
- Work out the route that the participant needs to take in relation to the goals identified in the first session.
- Look at the time that it would take to use the bus to get to a set location.
- Go to the bus shelter and look at the bus shelter timetable.
- Having made sure that the participant has sufficient money for the fare, model how you would go about hailing and riding the bus, and exiting the bus.
- This exercise will probably need to be repeated several times.

Session 3: Library – internet public transport website

- Arrange to visit the public library.
- Access the computers at the library and show the participant how to access the internet.
- Access the internet translink site and look at the timetables.
- Decide on a route and time you need to access the bus.
- Arrange to go on a bus ride – have the participant independently hail the bus, apply for the fare and exit at the agreed location. If you think the participant needs support and encouragement, accompany him on the bus trip.

Session 4: Planning and scheduling

- Look at the days and times when the participant needs to go to his groups, appointments and shopping.
- Organise the bus timetable schedule.
- Get the participant to independently access this transport.
- Arrange to meet the participant at an agreed place to check that he has managed this task independently.
- This activity should be repeated several times until the participant is confident with accessing public transport by himself.

Cooking

The other issue that Sam had difficulty with was preparing meals so he has now been enrolled in a cooking programme, a follow-on programme from Food for Life (see Chapter 12). In the Food for Life programme, there is an emphasis on the food groups, a need for physical activity every day, being able to plan and buy meals, and budgeting for healthy eating. In each group session, there is revision of the food pyramid and of the Kilo Cent$ counter (addressed in Chapter 12). The actual food that is prepared depends on the choices made by the group participants. Recipes should go in folders that participants can take home but must bring back for each session. All group sessions follow a similar plan. The following sessions and food recipes are suggestions only. The group need to select their own themes, for example special occasions like birthdays, Valentines Day, Easter, and recipes that are nutritious, easy to prepare and are in keeping with whatever theme has been chosen. It is unlikely that people will have a well-equipped and spacious kitchen but the basic equipment, e.g knives, bowls, spoons, cutlery, plates, saucepans and baking dishes, should be available.

Cooking Up a Storm

This group programme focuses on the development of the following skills.

- Understand the basis of nutrition.
- Plan a daily menu that is nutritious and considers their food preferences.
- Budgeting for food purchases and learning shopping skills including comparative shopping and understanding food labels.
- Food preparation and hygiene (including hand washing, use of cooking utensils and storage of food).
- Learning to work as a team for the production of the meal.
- Social skills involved in sharing a meal.

The programme could be done individually but the person would not receive the benefit of interaction with others.

Recipes for this programme could be collected from the internet, recipe books or magazines. They could even be family recipes that have been handed down. It is important for people to have a copy of the recipe to take away with them as it is more likely that they will cook the food again if they can access the recipe easily.

Session 1: Introduction

- Warm-up activity: using pictures of food, revise the food pyramid (see Chapter 12) by having participants place the food on the pyramid where they belong.
- Explain the purpose and goals of Cooking Up a Storm. Explain that the group will be shopping, preparing the food, eating and cleaning up after the meal.
- Have participants identify themes for each of the following sessions, e.g. winter meal, summer meal, special occasion, international, etc. Once themes have been decided by the group, they then select recipes for the following week including either an entrée or dessert and a main meal. These recipes are kept in folders which the participants can take home.
- Cooldown: revise the Kilo Cent$ counter (in Chapter 12) and how to compare prices and how to read nutritional lists.

Session 2: Winter

Irish stew and bread rolls.

- Warm-up activity: prepare shopping list.
- Review where all food items sit on the food pyramid.
- Go shopping and while shopping, use the Kilo Cent$ counter (see Chapter 12) to assist in making appropriate purchases.
- Return to kitchen. Form working teams to complete each food item. The bread rolls will have been purchased. Prepare food and eat. Between courses, consider how much was spent and how that fits with the 10-part shopping plan (see Chapter 12).
- Clean up. Revise theme and recipes for next week.

Session 3: Summer

Grilled chicken and salad followed by citrus pie.
Refer to the instructions for session 2.

Session 4: Birthday dinner

Minestrone soup followed by roast vegetables and a leg of lamb.
Refer to the instructions for session 2.

Session 5: International

Middle Eastern bread and dips followed by rogan josh.
Refer to the instructions for session 2.

Session 6: Vegetarian

Vegetarian lasagne followed by custard and fruit.
Refer to the instructions for session 2.

Session 7: Brunch

Fresh fruit followed by an English breakfast.
Refer to the instructions for session 2.

Session 8: Hamburger day

Hamburger followed by jelly and ice-cream.
Refer to the instructions for session 2.

Session 9: Graduation

Chicken soup followed by baked fish with chips and salad followed by sticky date pudding.

- Warm-up activity: prepare shopping list.
- Review where all food items sit on the food pyramid.
- Go shopping and while shopping, use the Kilo Cent$ counter (see Chapter 12) to assist in making appropriate purchases.
- Return to kitchen. Form working teams to complete each food item. The bread rolls will have been purchased. Prepare food and eat. Between courses, consider how much was spent and how that fits with the 10-part shopping plan (see Chapter 12).
- Clean up.
- Wish people all the best in continuing with this programme in the future.

Table 13.1 lists examples of budget recipes that could be used in the group. The recipes are for four people so the ingredients may need to be increased depending on how many people you have in the group. Of course, when planning the menus to use, it is necessary to consider the cultural group you are working with, if there are any dietary restrictions, e.g. Muslims do not eat pork, or whether there are vegetarians in the group.

Table 13.1   Sample menus: cooking on a shoestring.

Recipe	Method
Session 1: Easy potato bake	
Ingredients:	Preheat oven to 180°C.
4 potatoes, sliced	In a greased ovenproof dish, spread a layer of
250 g diced bacon	potatoes over the base.
4 tomatoes, sliced	Add slices of tomato, diced onion, bacon,
300 ml cream	cream and a handful of cheese.
1 cup grated cheese	Sprinkle on salt and pepper
Salt and pepper	Continue until the dish is full, finishing with a
	generous layer of cheese on the top.
	Cook in a moderate oven until potatoes are soft
	and the top is golden brown.
	This will take approximately 45–50 minutes.
	Serve with a green salad.
Session 2: Beef burgers	
Ingredients:	Mix everything in a bowl. Add salt and pepper.
500 g low-fat mince	Shape into 4 large balls.
1 onion, diced finely	Place in a hot, oiled pan and press flat (about
1 carrot, grated	2–3 cm thick) with spatula.
1 egg, beaten	Cook each side until they are done all the way
Salt and pepper	through.
	Serve on hamburger rolls with lettuce, tomato
	and beetroot.
Session 3: Spaghetti	
Ingredients:	Cook onion in olive oil until golden brown.
500 g low-fat mince	Add garlic.
1 onion, finely chopped	Add mince, capsicum (pepper) and parsley and
1 capsicum (pepper), diced	cook until mince is done.
Fresh parsley, chopped	Sprinkle in salt and pepper.
2 cloves garlic, crushed	Add the spaghetti sauce and simmer.
Premade pasta sauce	Bring a pot of water to the boil and add
Salt and pepper	spaghetti and cook until ready (al dente).
½ × 500 g spaghetti or other pasta of your	Serve with garlic bread and an Italian salad.
choice	Sprinkle with parmesan cheese.
Parmesan cheese	
Session 4: Meatloaf	
Ingredients:	Preheat the oven to 200°C.
500 g low-fat mince	Combine the mince, onion, carrot, egg and salt
1 onion, finely diced	and pepper.
1 carrot, grated	Place the ingredients into a greased loaf tin
1 egg, beaten	(rectangular).
Cheese, grated	Place grated cheese on top.
Salt and pepper	Bake in a moderate oven (180°C) for
	approximately 45 minutes.
	Serve with vegetables such as potato, beans,
	broccoli, sweet potato, etc.
Session 5: Tuna, pea and potato cakes	
Ingredients:	Place potatoes in a pot of cold water.
500 g potatoes, peeled and diced	Bring to the boil and cook for approximately
½ cup frozen baby peas	15 minutes or until tender.
415 g can tuna, drained and flaked	Bring peas to the boil, approximately 10 minutes.

Table 13.1   *(cont'd)*

Recipe	Method
2 tablespoons chopped fresh dill 1 egg lightly beaten ⅓ cup plain flour ⅓ cup vegetable oil Salt and pepper Mixed salad and lemon wedges to serve	Mash the potato. Add tuna, dill, peas and egg to the mash. Add salt and pepper. Stir to combine. Shape mixture into 8 patties. Coat patties in flour and refrigerate for 30 minutes. Heat oil in a frying pan and cook patties approximately 4 minutes or until golden. Serve with salad and lemon wedges.

Session 6: Sausage, egg and vegetable pie

Ingredients:	
1 onion, chopped finely 6 thin beef sausages 1 carrot, peeled and grated 2 zucchini (courgettes), grated 1 cup grated tasty cheese ½ cup plain flour 1½ cups milk 3 eggs Salt and pepper	Preheat the oven to 180°C. Cook onion until softened. Remove and place in a bowl. Add sausages to pan and cook until cooked through. Set aside for approximately 10 minutes, and then thinly slice. Place sausages, onion, carrot, zucchini and cheese in a prepared dish. Add salt and pepper. Whisk flour and milk in a bowl until smooth. Add eggs and whisk to combine. Pour over sausage mixture. Bake in a moderate oven for 50–60 minutes or until set. Serve with salad.

Session 7: Chilli con carne

Ingredients:	
125 g diced bacon 750 g lean beef mince 2 onions, finely chopped 2 medium red capsicums (peppers), chopped 3 garlic cloves, crushed 1 teaspoon chilli 2 tablespoons tomato paste 800 g diced tinned tomato 400 g red kidney beans, drained and rinsed Salt and pepper	Cook mince for approximately 15 minutes or until browned. Add bacon and cook. Add onion, capsicum (pepper), garlic and chilli and cook until softened. Add tomatoes, paste and 1 cup water, salt and pepper. Simmer for approximately 30 minutes. Add beans and cook for 15 minutes. Serve with steamed rice and jalapeno chillies, sour cream, chopped coriander leaves and grated tasty cheese as toppings.

Session 8: Chickpea curry

Ingredients:	
1 tin chickpeas 1 tin diced tomatoes 1 onion, finely chopped 1 dessert spoon grated ginger 2 cloves garlic, crushed 1 teaspoon turmeric 2 teaspoons coriander 1 teaspoon cumin Salt and pepper	Add chopped onion to pan and fry until lightly browned. Add garlic, ginger, turmeric, coriander, cumin and salt and pepper to taste. Stir for a minute or two then add chickpeas and tomatoes. Cook for 15 minutes over a moderate heat. Serve with rice and salad and mango chutney.

(continued)

Table 13.1   (cont'd)

Recipe	Method
Session 9: Stuffed zucchini (courgettes)	
Ingredients:	Preheat the oven to 180°C.
4 large zucchinis (courgettes)	Brush oven tray with oil.
1 onion, finely chopped	Cut the zucchini (courgettes) in half lengthways.
250 g diced bacon	Using a small spoon, scoop out the flesh.
2 garlic cloves, crushed	Dice the flesh.
300 g mince	Heat oil in pan, add onion, bacon and garlic
1½ cups cooked rice	until lightly browned.
1 cup tomato puree	Add the mince and cook until well done.
1 teaspoon dried mixed herbs	Add rice, tomato puree, chilli, herbs, salt and
Salt and pepper	pepper and chopped zucchini (courgettes).
½ teaspoon chilli powder	Cook for a few minutes.
2 tablespoons parmesan cheese	Spoon the mixture into the zucchini (courgette) shells, sprinkle with cheese.
	Place on the prepared oven tray and bake for approximately 30 minutes.
	Serve with mashed potato and tomato slices.

There are basic principles that should underpin the selection of recipes for menus. These include such things as:

- low-cost ingredients
- readily available to purchase
- high nutritional value
- preparation possible without using sophisticated equipment
- simple preparation steps
- food that people enjoy eating.

Summary

After attending the rehabilitation programme, Sam is now able to catch the bus independently, is managing his finances better and has found some recipes that he enjoys cooking. He is feeling much better about himself now that he is able to take care of himself more effectively. Sam will need to have follow-up to see if he is actually able to do cooking activities at home. Home visits could be arranged and a plan made for Sam to cook something for this visit.

   After some discussion with Sam, you realise that he now would like to find work so you refer him to the vocational rehabilitation programme. It must be remembered that building confidence and skill is a slow process. Motivation is also an issue when it is so much easier to buy fast food. People with severe mental illness and who are in the low-income bracket tend to have diets higher in fat and refined sugars and lower in fibre than the general population. There is also the tendency to have an inadequate amount of fruit and vegetable intake and a tendency to drink carbonated drinks rather than water.

Acknowledgements

Chris Lloyd and Hazel Bassett worked for Rehabilitation Services, Gold Coast Health Service District at the time that these programmes were developed.

Resources

http://www.taste.com.au/recipes/collections/budget
http://allrecipes.co.uk/recipes/budget-recipes.apsx
www.taste.com.au
http://www.taste.com.au/recipes/colllections/quick+meals
http://allrecipes.com.au
www.cookdinner.com
www.recipes.com.au
http://recipefinder.ninemsn.com.au
www.cuisine.com.au
www.goodrecipes.com.au
http://www.lifestylefood.com.au/recipes/collections/mince-recipes.aspx
http://www.taste.com.au/recipes/collections/chicken
http://www.taste.com.au/recipes/collections/beef+recipes
http://www.taste.com.au/recipes/collections/lamb+recipes
http://www.taste.com.au/recipes/collections/vegetarian

Part IV
Peer Support and Self-Help

Chapter 14

Peer Support in a Mental Health Service Context

Lindsay Oades, Frank P. Deane and Julie Anderson

Introduction

This chapter will first summarise the range of definitions that have been provided for peer support, in a mental health context. Clarifications of the different aims of peer support initiatives and the potential psychological processes that underpin them are then provided. Three key forms that peer support groups may take are then described and we track Sam as he experiences peer support in the context of job seeking. A summary of existing empirical evidence for peer support groups is provided before examining some of the necessary tensions that may exist between the alternative views of those coming from inside the consumer/survivor/ex-patient (c/s/x) movement perspective, and the traditional discourses based on the medical approach. A series of recommendations is then offered for those who are working or about to work within a peer support framework in mental health. The recommendations include things to do and things to avoid.

Definitions of peer support

There are several ways to conceptualise peer support. The working definition for this chapter is a process of mutual support where persons voluntarily come together to help each other address common problems or shared concerns (Davidson *et al.*, 2006). Solomon (2004) defines peer support as 'social emotional support, frequently coupled with instrumental support, that is mutually offered or provided by persons having a mental health condition to others sharing a similar mental health condition to bring about a desired social or personal change' (p.393).

Moreover, the participation in this process is usually intentional, and the social context enables the person to find resources and structures that enhance their ability to deal with problems and concerns.

Adame and Leitner (2008) explain that the medical model underemphasises issues such as social conditions, political oppression, family systems, interpersonal relationships,

Manual of Psychosocial Rehabilitation, First Edition. Edited by Robert King, Chris Lloyd, Tom Meehan, Frank P. Deane and David J. Kavanagh.
© 2012 Blackwell Publishing Ltd. Published 2012 by Blackwell Publishing Ltd.

spiritual crises and the trauma of physical and sexual abuse that are experienced by many people seeking help. In contrast, the peer support model is based on the premise that significant interpersonal relationships and a sense of community provide a context for personal recovery and empowerment.

One important distinction within approaches to peer support is those groups that generally accept the overall mental health system, and seek to work to reform it, improve it and assist consumers to have more choices within this system. Those who identify more with the survivor/ex-patient philosophy will more likely seek alternatives outside the system. This distinction can be thought of as two different discourses: the medical discourse of symptoms and 'objectivity' versus a discourse related to individual suffering situated within social and political environments that often include oppression and injustice. It has been asserted that 'peer support ... becomes a natural extension and expansion of community rather than modeling professionalized caretaking of people defined as defective' (Mead *et al.*, 2001, p.136). There is usually a greater expectancy of reciprocity in the relationship between peer support workers and those they work with compared to more 'expert' professional workers.

Whilst peer support definitely includes emotional healing as a result of shared interpersonal experiences, psychiatric survivors and ex-patients will often adopt a more politically oriented definition of empowerment that emphasises political activism and advocacy work to an equal if not greater extent than individual peer support (Crossley & Crossley, 2001; Everett, 2000). Several authors have described how peer support groups foster alternative views of the meaning of recovery which may be more about recovering from iatrogenic trauma than mental illness itself. For example, the stigma associated with mental illness, and the consequent disadvantage and disenfranchisement experienced by those with mental illness, may be an important theme within a group of peers. An important component of peer support lies in understanding that it occurs in a political context and is a social process.

Forms of peer support initiatives

There are several schemes that have been used to describe the different forms that peer support initiatives can take. Using the foci of groups described by Cohen and Mullender (2005), peer support groups can be classified as:

* *remedial*, focusing on the personal processes of recovery
* *interactional*, emphasising the interpersonal relationships and personal experience
* *social*, integrating the personal, interpersonal and political. The social classification involves social change and empowerment.

Solomon (2004) describes processes underpinning peer support as social support, experiential knowledge, helper–therapy principle, social learning theory and social comparison. Groups can also vary in how conservative or radical they are with regard to their level of political activism (Solomon, 2004).

Davidson *et al.* (2009) suggest that there are three forms that peer support groups may take: naturally occurring mutual support groups, consumer-run services, and the employment

---

Box14.1   Terms used to describe peer support initiatives

Consumer-delivered services (Salzer & Shear, 2002)
Consumer drop-in centres (Mowbray *et al.*, 2002)
Consumer-operated self-help centres (Swarbrick, 2007)
Consumer-run businesses (Kimura *et al.*, 2002)
Consumer-run services (Goldstrom *et al.*, 2006)
Consumer-run organisations (Clay *et al.*, 2005)
Consumer/survivor initiatives (Nelson *et al.*, 2001)
Mutual-help groups (Corrigan *et al.*, 2005)
Mutual support groups (Chien *et al.*, 2008)
Self-help agencies (Segal & Silverman, 2002)
Self-development programmes (Oades *et al.*, 2009)
Self-help programmes (Chamberlin *et al.*, 1996)

---

of consumers as providers within clinical and rehabilitative settings. Employment of consumers as providers within clinical and rehabilitative settings in many ways is a product of system change from the original activism. Across these three broad forms, many specific terms have been used to describe peer support initiatives, as illustrated in Box 14.1.

Peer support programmes can sit within traditional community-based psychosocial rehabilitation services as a peer partnership model. This means they give up some control of legal, financial and content of the programme (Solomon, 2004).

Peer support sits on a continuum of helping relationships. On the continuum are unidirectional intentional relationships, with professionals and peers in service settings, reciprocal relationships such as reciprocal groups facilitated by peers as providers of conventional services, to naturally occurring reciprocal relationships with peers in community/and or service settings (Davidson *et al.*, 2006).

Sam's experiences of peer support

Sam is very committed to getting a job. He is assigned an employment consultant to work with him on individual placement and support. This is an example of a unidirectional relationship with a professional in a service setting. Sam's confidence in gaining work is low because of his past employment history. The employment consultant suggests that Sam meet regularly with a peer mentor, employed by the service (unidirectional intentional relationship with a peer). Sam continues to meet the employment consultant and the peer mentor. The peer mentor shares her experience in gaining employment and the issues and strategies for working with a mental illness. The employment consultant works on needs assessment, goal setting and goal attainment with Sam and the peer mentor, as a team.

The peer mentor suggests an 8-week peer education course around recovery developed and facilitated by peers employed by the service (reciprocal groups facilitated by peers as providers). In the peer education course, Sam meets other people with similar experiences to himself whilst they work as a peer group on issues such as dealing with stigma, medication, personal treatment strategies, consumer rights and communication. At the completion of the course, Sam has made new friendships, feels confident to update his skills, and has renewed hope in looking for work.

Eventually Sam gains part-time employment. The peer mentor suggests to Sam that he may wish to attend employment dinners with other people who work and have a mental illness. The employment dinners are supported by the psychosocial rehabilitation service and are peer run (self-help mutual support, intentional, voluntary reciprocal relationships). Sam meets other people with similar interests and they decide to go to the pictures on a regular basis (friendship, naturally occurring reciprocal relationships).

Necessary tensions in peer support contexts

We use the phrase 'necessary tension' to capture the political essence of many peer support initiatives. One ongoing tension relates to payment for peer support workers. As Crossley (2004) explains, the trend for members of the c/s/x movement to be sought out and paid for their expertise is a double-edged sword: 'At one level this is a victory for the movement. However, as some consultants and activists recognize, it changes the modus operandi of the movement in significant and not always desirable ways. A political model is replaced by a business model' (p.176). However, many may argue that the situation is less polarised than this. A peer support employee can have a position description that includes strong advocacy and organisational change. This may be outside the original view of early advocates within the c/s/x movement but may still generate major system transformation.

A further key issue relates to concerns of existing staff members who do not identify as peers. Some mental health professionals may feel concerned about peer support workers for a range of reasons, including reduced productivity, increased risk or simply having their own jobs replaced. An alternative view is that peer support workers are additional resources who will help divert the overload of clients from already overworked mental health professionals (Solomon, 2004; Solomon & Draine, 2001).

In the partnership model, consumers (who have psychiatric diagnoses) partner with mental health professionals (who do not have psychiatric diagnoses) in the co-ordination and delivery of services. Everett (2000) cautions against aspects of partnership models, asserting that those in marginalised positions of power can try to exert their influence on partnership models but their voices will never carry the same weight as mental health professionals 'because the powerful retain exclusive rights over the definition of what is and is not "normal"' (p.164).

As the employment of peer support workers increases within mental health services, the partnership model may take on added complexity or possibly lose its original meaning. Whilst there is a service provider and a service user, the issue of whether the service provider identifies as having used a mental health service or experienced a mental illness may become subsumed as one type of expertise, i.e. lived experience complementing professional training (Blanch *et al.*, 1993).

Summary of evidence from peer support programmes

The traditional empirical approach with the randomised experimental design seen as the highest standard of evidence may be of little value to many involved in peer support initiatives. This again is part of the necessary tension that occurs, and is yet another example of the differences between the medical paradigm, which places great importance on 'objectivity', and a c/s/x perspective which highly values subjective personal experiences and context.

The empirical literature on peer support consists largely of quasi-experimental studies, qualitative reports and anecdotal accounts of innovative programmes, as opposed to randomised trials. There has been a systematic review of empirical studies that assessed whether participating in mutual help groups for mental health problems leads to improved psychological and social functioning (Pistrang *et al.*, 2010). The 12 studies that met the criteria provided limited but promising evidence that mutual help groups benefit people with three types of problems: chronic mental illness, depression/ anxiety and bereavement. These authors report that five of the 12 studies demonstrated no differences in mental health outcomes between mutual help group members and non-members. None of the studies showed evidence of negative effects. The studies varied greatly in terms of design quality and more high-quality outcome research is needed.

Repper and Carter (2011) reviewed research on peers offering support for people with mental health problems working from professionally led mental health services (e.g. statutory or public services). They located seven randomised controlled trials that described a wide range of peer support work interventions – for example, peers employed as case managers, additional to team members, in outpatient and inpatient services. They reported 'inconsistent findings' across studies due to highly variable outcome measures. However, the most consistent finding appeared to be that those services using peer support workers demonstrated a reduction in hosptial admissions and longer community tenure amongst those consumers or mental health services with whom they worked. A range of other benefits were reported from either single studies or qualitative studies. These included a greater sense of independence and empowerment, improved social functioning, feeling more accepted, understood and liked, experiencing stigma as less of a barrier to employment. There were also multiple benefits reported for the peer support workers themselves (e.g. personal growth, esteem).

The evidence base for peer support in mental health services is growing but there is a need for organisational studies. That is, it is not sufficient to conceptualise peer support initiatives only at the individual level and assess the benefits and psychological functioning of the individual. Peer support initiatives should also be investigated as to how they lead to organisational transformation of culture, and how they interface with the policy related to recovery-oriented service provision (Slade *et al.*, 2008).

The following is a brief example of a peer support service provided by a psychosocial rehabilitation service in Australia that attempts to addresses some of the organisational issues that arise.

Example of a peer support service

The example is set in a psychosocial rehabilitation service that incorporates peer support services. The service established a consumer participation unit (CPU) which broadly aimed to facilitate communication and understanding of the lived experience of mental illness in the context of traditional service provision. Staff who have experienced mental illness were employed. Their role was to facilitate community participation, participation within the organisation and participation by individuals with their own healthcare planning. The role of the unit in the organisation was to inform and support the organisation on consumer issues. A specific example of activity facilitated by the CPU was the establishment of and support for a speaker's bureau of peers to educate the community and staff on issues to do with having a mental illness. The CPU trains and supports peers to facilitate an 8-week peer education course. The unit co-trains staff on rehabilitation practices. It works with day programmes to incorporate peer programmes within traditional service offerings. It also aims to bring the latest evidence and practice on peer support and consumer issues to the organisation within a recovery framework.

Recommendations regarding implementation of peer support initiatives

In their review, Repper and Carter (2011) identified a number of challenges in peer support work. These challenges include multiple *boundary* issues such as being perceived as more of a friend to service users as a result of sharing personal information and experiences. *Power* issues emerge as a result of peer workers being formally employed with all of the associated benefits, thus potentially elevating their status in relation to the consumers they work with. Similarly, they may be viewed as 'patients' by other professional staff with whom they work, undermining their status. *Stress* has been identified as a potential challenge since it could result in recurrence of mental health problems. Worry about this concern may mean that fewer demands are placed on peer support workers by line management, which may limit the roles they are able to play in the service. The final challenge identified involves maintaining a *distinct role* for peer support workers. This issue intersects with the 'necessary tensions' noted above in that consumers need to maintain the principles associated with recovery-oriented practices and take care not to be socialised into the traditional way of working in mental health services.

In this final section, the aim is to provide recommendations to those who aim to commence peer support groups or improve those already under way. These recommendations address a number of the challenges noted. Below a set of prescriptions (things to do) and proscriptions (things to avoid) are provided, written predominantly in the context of peer groups within or attached to a mental health system.

Prescriptions

1. *Clarify early and gain input from a range of people about the primary focus of groups.* That is, are they *remedial*, focusing on the personal processes of recovery, *interactional*, emphasising the interpersonal relationships and personal experience, or *social*, integrating the personal, interpersonal and political, which the authors refer to as social change and empowerment of oppressed populations?
2. *Clarify early and gain input from a range of people as to the advantages and disadvantages of each of the three main forms of peer support.* That is, are they naturally occurring

mutual support groups, consumer-run services, or the employment of consumers as providers within clinical and rehabilitative settings? It is also important to remember that any larger service may have a combination of these types of groups. Explicitly clarify the continuum of peer and non-peer involvement across the agency.

3. *Systematically seek to create 'buy-in' or ownership for peer services from all parts of the organisation.* This can be in the form of presentations at all staff forums and allocated time at staff meetings for personal stories on the effect of peer support. Strategies that embed peer support include establishing work procedures and practices that reflect the values of peer support as an effective psychosocial rehabilitation offering; suitable training and support for peer workers, facilitators and educators; and implementation of peer supervision for peer workers. Strategies require realistic timelines for change to have the greatest opportunity to be embedded and succeed. Organisational change models should be considered.

4. *Use external influences including research, presentations of international best practice, organisational visits, etc.* As outlined previously, whilst the discourse of many peer support initiatives is personal and political rather than medical, this in no way means they should not have the same rigour and scholarship supporting them. Some aspects of peer support groups may be similar to communities of practice or journal clubs, which include the sharing of ideas, personal and other. In the USA, consumer and consumer-supporter national technical assistance centres have been established to support such processes (Rogers, 2010).

5. *Set up organisational structures that allow discussion of the 'necessary tensions' associated with peer support work.* For example, members of a peer support group may question and explore difficulties with medical prescriptions. Hence, if a peer support worker is employed by a clinical agency, in this regard it would make little sense for them to be operationally reporting to a treating doctor. Whilst the individuals involved may manage the tension well, organisational structures, e.g. lines of reporting, should be designed to allow these tensions to be addressed.

6. *As a general philosophy, aim to keep groups and practices semi-structured, autonomous, non-hierarchical and non-bureaucratic.* This provides a challenge for many health services with their emphasis on quality or evidence base. They are not, however, necessarily opposing. Quality service provision and effective service provision do not necessarily require an *a priori* fully structured programme. They are more likely to involve useful processes that have worked elsewhere that require tailoring to the context at hand.

7. *Examine ways for your agency to link with state, national and international efforts to certify and accredit peer specialists.* Well-managed organisations will already be aware of policy initiatives in this regard and seek to align their workforce and workforce development in line with these principles.

8. *Develop research programmes around the peer support initiatives, particularly using methods and approaches consistent with the peer support movement.* For example, participatory action research and qualitative methods will probably be consistent with the aims and philosophy of many within peer support groups. These, however, are rigorous methods and will require technical support in the same way quantitative methods often require consultants to support them.

Proscriptions

1. *Do not use clinical staff members who have been with the service for many years to now lead peer support initiatives.* This would be neither peer led nor likely to lead to system transformation aligned with peer support values.
2. *Do not employ peer support workers solely because they cost less at the moment than clinically trained staff members.* Whilst in the short term this may provide a useful strategy for having a greater number of peer support workers within a service, in the longer term it is not consistent with the non-hierarchical philosophy of not privileging one discourse over another.
3. *Do not think of peer support initiatives simply as groups.* Peer support is a multifaceted phenomenon that may be spontaneous or planned. It may occur in a formal group setting or may represent an overarching culture underpinning the ongoing evolution of recovery-oriented service provision. Health services should avoid viewing this solely as a personal or interpersonal process, and think of it also as a service and organisational transformational process, and also accept that much of it is occurring and will occur outside the service system.

Summary

This chapter has provided an overview of key issues in peer support at a time when awareness and policy regarding peer support initiatives are growing in many western nations. Key recommendations have been provided about how to develop or improve peer support initiatives. We have argued for structures and processes to maintain the 'necessary tension' between some of the philosophies stemming from the c/s/x movement that has underpinned peer support work with the traditional medical models that have dominated mental health service provision.

References

Adame AL, Leitner LM (2008) Breaking out of the mainstream: the evolution of peer support alternatives to the mental health system. *Ethical Human Psychology and Psychiatry* **10**, 146–62.
Blanch A, Fischer D, Tucker W, Walsh D, Chassman J (1993) Consumer practitioners and psychiatrists share insights about recovery and coping. *Disability Studies Quarterly* **13**, 17–20.
Chamberlin J, Rogers E, Ellison ML (1996) Self-help programs: a description of their characteristics and their members. *Psychiatric Rehabilitation Journal* **19**, 33–42.
Chien WT, Thompson DR, Norman I (2008) Evaluation of a peer-led mutual support group for Chinese families of people with schizophrenia. *American Journal of Community Psychology* **42**, 122–34.
Clay S, Schell B, Corrigan PW, Ralph RO (2005) *On Our Own, Together: Peer Programs for People with Mental Illness.* Vanderbilt University Press: Nashville, TN.
Cohen MB, Mullender A (2005) The personal in the political: exploring the group work continuum from individual to social change goals. *Social Work with Groups* **28**, 187–204.
Corrigan PW, Slopen N, Gracia G, Phelan S, Keogh CB, Keck L (2005) Some recovery processes in mutual help groups for persons with mental illness; II: qualitative analysis of participant interviews. *Community Mental Health Journal* **41**, 721–35.

Crossley ML, Crossley N (2001) "Patient" voices, social movements and the habitus: how psychiatric survivors "speak out." *Social Science and Medicine* **52**, 1477–89.

Crossley N (2004) Not being mentally ill: social movements, system survivors and the oppositional habitus. *Anthropology Medicine* **11**, 161–80.

Davidson L, Chinman M, Sells D, Rowe M (2006) Peer support among adults with serious mental illness: a report from the field. *Schizophrenia Bulletin* **32**, 443–50.

Davidson L, Chinman M, Kloos B *et al.* (2009) Peer support among individuals with severe mental illness: a review of the evidence. *Clinical Psychology: Science and Practice* **6**, 165–87.

Everett B (2000) *A Fragile Revolution: Consumers and Psychiatric Survivors Confront the Power of the Mental Health System.* Wilfrid University Press: Waterloo, Canada.

Goldstrom ID, Campbell J, Rogers JA *et al.* (2006) National estimates for mental health mutual support groups, self-help organizations, and consumer-operated services. *Administration and Policy in Mental Health and Mental Health Services Research* **33**, 92–103.

Kimura M, Mukaiyachi I, Ito E (2002) The House of Bethel and consumer-run businesses: an innovative approach to psychiatric rehabilitation. *Canadian Journal of Community Mental Health* **21**, 69–77.

Mead S, Hilton D, Curtis L (2001) Peer support: a theoretical perspective. *Psychiatric Rehabilitation Journal* **25**, 134–41.

Mowbray CT, Robinson EA, Holter MC (2002) Consumer drop-in centers: operations, services, and consumer involvement. *Health and Social Work* **24**, 248–61.

Nelson G, Lord J, Ochocka J (2001) *Shifting the Paradigm in Community Mental Health: Towards Empowerment and Community.* University of Toronto Press: Toronto, Canada.

Oades LG, Andresen R, Crowe, TP, Malins GM, Andresen R, Turner A (2008) A Handbook to Flourish. *A Self-Development Program for People with Enduring Mental Illness.* Illawarra Institute for Mental Health, University of Wollongong: Wollongong, Australia.

Pistrang N, Barker C, Humphreys K (2010) The contributions of mutual help groups for mental health problems to psychological well-being: a systematic review. In: Brown LD, Wituk S (eds) *Mental Health Self-Help: Consumer and Family Initiatives.* Springer Verlag: New York, pp.61–86.

Repper J, Carter T (2011) A review of the literature on peer support in mental health services. *Journal of Mental Health* **20**(4), 392–411.

Rogers S (2010) Consumer and consumer-supporter national technical assistance centers: helping the consumer movement grow and transform systems. In: Brown LD, Wituk S (eds) *Mental Health Self-Help: Consumer and Family Initiatives.* Springer Verlag: New York, pp.265–86.

Salzer MS, Shear SL (2002) Identifying consumer-provider benefits in evaluations of consumer-delivered services. *Psychiatric Rehabilitation Journal* **25**, 281–8.

Segal SP, Silverman C (2002) Determinants of client outcomes in self-help agencies. *Psychiatric Services* **53**, 304–9.

Slade M, Amering M, Oades L (2008) Recovery: an international perspective. *Epidemiologia e Psichiatria Sociale* **17**, 128–37.

Solomon P (2004) Peer support/peer provided services underlying processes, benefits, and critical ingredients. *Psychiatric Rehabilitation Journal* **27**, 392–401.

Solomon P, Draine J (2001) The state of knowledge of the effectiveness of consumer provided services. *Psychiatric Rehabilitation Journal* **25**, 20–7.

Swarbrick M (2007) Consumer-operated self-help centers. *Psychiatric Rehabilitation Journal* **31**, 76–9.

Chapter 15

Supporting Families and Carers

Robert King and Trevor Crowe

Introduction

This chapter provides guidance for practitioners that will assist them to support families and carers with a family member or friend affected by severe mental illness. It begins by identifying some of the components of burden of care for families and then provides recommendations regarding provision of psychoeducation, collaboration with families in provision of services and recovery support. It also describes the use of problem-solving and strengths-focused techniques to assist families to manage challenges associated with care, as well as orient them towards their own personal and relational empowerment. The chapter concludes with a section that outlines the benefits of support provided by peers and provides links to some peer support resources.

> Sam's mother has been feeling down lately. It has become clear to her that Sam is not going to make a quick recovery and that he may not lead the same life that others in his age group seem to effortlessly move into – higher education, work, marriage. She alternates between feeling sad and worried that she might have done something or not done something when he was younger and feeling frustrated and angry that he is not getting on with his life. She also feels exasperated with the mental health services. She knows they are trying to help but she doesn't understand what they are doing with Sam or why he is not getting better.

Burden of care

There is no doubt that family members and sometimes friends often experience burden of care when trying to support a relative or friend with a severe mental illness such as schizophrenia. This burden can be compounded when co-occurring disorders such as substance abuse are present. By burden, we mean that providing care is experienced as emotionally demanding and stressful over an extended period. Carers have been found to exhibit very

Manual of Psychosocial Rehabilitation, First Edition. Edited by Robert King, Chris Lloyd, Tom Meehan, Frank P. Deane and David J. Kavanagh.
© 2012 Blackwell Publishing Ltd. Published 2012 by Blackwell Publishing Ltd.

low wellbeing as a result of the demands of care giving (Cummins *et al.*, 2007). Carers report a range of psychological problems such as depression, anxiety and stress (Briggs & Fisher, 2000; Butler & Bauld, 2005). Carers also often report financial burden, having less time for themselves, and negative impacts of illness and stigma on relationships (Kirby *et al.*, 1999; Milliken & Nortcott, 2003; Ranganathan, 2004). Therefore, burden is not just about immediate stress related to care, but includes relational and personal disempowerment. Burden may be associated with one or more of the following.

- *Guilt* – feelings of responsibility for having contributed to the mental illness through inadequate parenting or partnering, through failure to seek help sufficiently early or to provide effective care. Guilt is often associated with feelings of inadequacy and personal failure. People respond to guilt differently. Some become depressed, whereas others project their guilt and blame others.
- *Fatigue* – feeling a lack of emotional strength or having insufficient resources to continue providing care. These may be associated with constant worry about the person with a mental illness, a sense of never being able to escape from care responsibilities, and the uncertainty of the illness trajectory or their own future.
- *Frustration* – these feelings may be directed towards the person with the mental illness, towards the health system or both. When directed towards the person with mental illness, the feeling may be that they are not trying to help themselves or are self-centred and unappreciative. When directed towards the health system, the feeling may be that the system is chaotic or disorganised, uncaring, that they let carers down or neglect them, or that it is plain incompetent.

The starting point for any effective work supporting families is understanding and respecting the burden of care. Effective work aims to reduce the burden and orient carers towards their own personal and relational empowerment. In turn, this work improves the likelihood that the person with the mental illness will feel supported in their recovery. Empowerment begets empowerment, which is central to recovery.

When symptoms are less prominent, acute episodes less frequent and life functioning more independent, burden is less. However, even when there is optimal treatment and rehabilitation, many people with severe conditions such as schizophrenia will continue to experience symptoms and impairments and it is in these circumstances that work supporting families is most effective and necessary.

When we are effective in reducing the burden on families, there are likely to be benefits for the client. There is good research evidence that when families and carers can reduce their burden, their interactions with the client are less entangled, enmeshed or conflictual, potentially more empowering, and are associated with reduced frequency of acute relapse (Barrowclough *et al.*, 2005; Clark, 2001; Glynn *et al.*, 2006; Moore, 2005; Schofield *et al.*, 2001; Needle *et al.*, 1988).

Carer burden can affect the carer's life to such an extent that they are in need of their own recovery. An obstacle here, though, is that carers will often view 'recovery' as only applicable to the person with the illness, only seeking help to manage the illness of the client and focusing on strategies to cope with the illness. This is to be expected, particularly in the earlier stages of the illness, as the person with the illness often becomes the central focus for the rest of the family, often drawing attention away from the needs and wants of other family members. This preoccupation can result in being enmeshed with the family member with the illness (e.g. Needle *et al.*, 1988) and an erosion of the other family members/carers' sense of self. It can have negative effects on their own wellbeing and growth (Schlesinger & Horberg, 1994). It is also not unusual for some family members to feel like they have lost contact with themselves completely (Karp & Tanarugsachock, 2000). If family members/carers are able to refocus back on themselves and their own experiences (Brown & Lewis, 1999; Muhlbauer, 2002), they are more likely to create a more positive self-image which helps them to more effectively negotiate the uncertainty of living with mental illness (Schlesinger & Horberg, 1994).

The skilled practitioner pursues ways of engaging carers such that they:

- feel heard
- have their experiences normalised where possible
- are provided with information and strategies to cope with the illness
- start to consider ways in which they could reconnect with their strengths
- take their own lives back
- find ways to move forward regardless of the fluctuations in illness symptomatology.

In effect, this type of personal and relational empowerment parallels personal recovery in mental illness (Buckley-Walker *et al.*, 2010; Slade *et al.*, 2008). If carers learn to help themselves they are in a better position to help the person with the illness.

Over recent years there has been an increasing focus on 'family recovery' (Karp & Tanarugsachock, 2000; Milliken & Nortcott, 2003; Muhlbauer, 2002; Pagnini, 2005; Rose *et al.*, 2002). Key family recovery stages emerging from this literature are:

- initial recognition of a problem (i.e. something is wrong but hoping it will just go away, yet preoccupation with client continues to build)
- clearer recognition or confirmation of a disorder, yet still hoping for a cure
- coming to terms with the chronicity/trajectory of illness
- acceptance of the illness, reclaiming one's own life.

Each of these stages requires different types of support for the family.

As outlined below, families and carers will probably benefit from accurate and practical information about illness features, origins and potential trajectories, particularly across the first three stages of family recovery. However, this recovery journey for families involves grief and loss, a reconfiguration of life directions, and working on personal and relational empowerment. This means the practitioner needs to be sensitive to where the individual family members may be on their journeys and what they are ready to work with, help them to feel heard and validated where they are, and help create opportunities for them to feel strong enough to move forward with their own lives.

There are six key ways in which we can contribute to reducing burden of care and increasing empowerment.

1. Psychoeducation
2. Collaboration and relational empowerment
3. Peer support

4. Problem solving
5. Strengths and values clarification
6. Goal setting and action planning

In this chapter we will look more closely at the three key interventions that are not covered in detail in other chapters, namely psychoeducation, collaboration and relational empowerment, and peer support. Please see Chapter 7 for more details and practical guidance as to how to work effectively with problem solving, strengths and values clarification, and goal setting and action planning.

Psychoeducation

Psychoeducation involves the provision of information about the person's illness and the potential effects on other family members. The central questions in the minds of most carers will be:

- How did it come about (and was it my fault)?
- Will she or he get better?
- What can I do to help?
- What might I do that is not helpful?

Carers will not always ask these questions directly, which means that it is the responsibility of the practitioner to address them, even if they are not raised. You can approach these topics by saying something like 'you might be wondering how or why he developed this illness' or 'people in your position often ask what the future holds for her'. Most times the carer will affirm that they do want information in the area you have flagged.

There are two broad approaches to psychoeducation, both of which have advantages and disadvantages. One approach is to communicate with the family from the position of an expert, whereas the other approach adopts a position of humility. You have to decide which suits the family better. If you are very skilled you can combine both but this can be difficult.

A position of expertise emphasises how much we now understand about mental illness, emphasising our understanding of its bioneurological basis and the power of evidence-based interventions, both psychopharmacological and psychosocial. The 'survival skills' workshops developed by Bill McFarlane and colleagues as a prelude to their multiple family psychoeducation group programme are a good example of this approach (McFarlane, 2004). Families are shown slides of brain scans that illustrate how schizophrenia is a disease of the brain and provided with high-quality information about the impact of antipsychotic medication. This kind of information is valuable because it builds confidence among families that the professional team in highly competent and up to date. It also imparts a very important message: schizophrenia is a brain disease and it is not your fault that your son or daughter has the misfortune to have acquired it.

In response to the first question listed above, the expert is likely to focus on the brain and to draw parallels with other conditions that involve constitutional defects of one or more organs. In other words, mental illness is caused by a brain defect or deficit. In response to the second question, the expert will focus on the importance of minimising relapse by careful compliance with medication, which regulates or compensates for the brain defect. In response to the third question, the expert will emphasise collaboration with the treating team, with the carer being a kind of ancillary case manager, looking out for early warning signs, monitoring medication compliance and supporting rehabilitation strategies. These are roles that many family members welcome (see below).

A position of humility emphasises how little we know about mental illness and its treatment. While acknowledging that a condition like schizophrenia involves disturbance of brain function, the humble practitioner equally admits that we have little understanding as to why or how some people develop the condition. With respect to medication, its value in treatment of acute episodes and prevention of future acute episodes is emphasised but it is equally acknowledged that there is little if any impact on negative symptoms and that side-effects such as weight gain are problematic and often difficult to manage. The humble practitioner is likely to emphasise recovery as a personal process and journey rather than something that is attributable to clinical interventions. The main advantage of humility is that family members do not develop unrealistic expectations. It may also reduce the risk of passivity. While the humble position does not so overtly absolve the family of any responsibility for the mental illness of a daughter or son, it avoids any kind of finger pointing.

In response to the first question, the humble practitioner will point to the complexity of causal factors, having reference to a biopsychosocial and/or stress diathesis model. In other words, while it is possible to point to a range of factors associated with mental illness, for any specific person it is difficult to be confident as to which or which combination of factors is most important. In response to the second question, the humble practitioner will point to evidence of a tendency for people to recover over time but will also highlight the variability of recovery trajectories and the difficulty of predicting which trajectory a particular person will take. In response to the third question, the humble practitioner might make some suggestions but also advocate for a trial and error or learning from experience approach – 'keep doing what works and stop doing what doesn't work'. It is also important, as mentioned above, that the humble practitioner recognises that each family member/carer has a unique recovery journey and may be more ready for some types of information and other interventions than other types. Adopting a curious, enquiring approach will help to determine the particular psychoeducational needs of the family member/carer.

Whatever position the practitioner adopts, it is useful to link families and carers seeking information to some of the many high-quality sources of information available online. It is also important to remember that simply pointing families and carers to information resources will not necessarily mean they will make the most of these resources, or in fact be able to access them. It is recommended that time is spent talking through key information with carers before providing them with written summaries and weblinks.

Some examples are:

- http://mentalhealth.com which is very good for information about diagnosis and treatment of different psychiatric disorders.
- http://www.sane.org which contains useful factsheets as well as some podcasts and other resources.

- http://www.rcpsych.ac.uk/mentalhealthinfoforall.aspx which provides factsheets and other resources prepared by the Royal College of Psychiatrists in the UK.
- http://www.arafmiaustralia.asn.au/recovery.html which provides useful information and stories of other people in relationship with people with mental illness.
- www.eppic.org.au Early Psychosis Prevention and Intervention Centre: information and fact sheets on psychosis.
- www.orygen.org.au ORYGEN specialist youth mental health service, a research centre and a range of education, training, advocacy and health promotion activities.
- www.mmha.org.au Multicultural Mental Health Australia: information about schizophrenia in different languages.

Relational empowerment

Another important psychoeducational area is that of unhelpful relationship dynamics, or reaction patterns, and how the carer might start to work on relational empowerment. As mentioned earlier, it is not unusual for different family members to deal with grief, loss and trauma in different ways. Recovery from mental illness or other problems like alcohol and drug abuse doesn't come with an instruction manual and families often take on roles that are understandable and driven by good intentions. However, sometimes these coping reactions can over time impede their own growth and the recovery of the person with the illness.

Some of the responses and roles carers adopt may be necessary at times. For example, when crisis occurs someone needs to take control. That person may take on the role of caretaker, peacemaker or rescuer. Other family members in the same situation might withdraw and start criticising what is going on from a distance. These reaction patterns may broadly fall under the roles of victim (where the carer feels their needs are not being met or are ignored), persecutor (where the carer is angry, fed up and critical) or rescuer (where the carer tries to fix everything, often driven by guilt and worry) (e.g. Choy, 1990; Fulkerson, 2003; Karpman, 1968). These roles usually have a function, such as easing tension or containing and trying to fix or change the 'problem'. It is important to know when certain reactions and roles are helpful and when they become less helpful. The main questions here are:

- Is the carer's behaviour helping themselves and the person with the illness, or is it taking responsibility for their recovery away from them?
- What is the function of the behaviour, and how might this function be better served?

An example of 'rescuing' might be keeping track of psychiatric medication and putting it out for the person with the illness to take. This may lead the person with the illness to feel complacency and/or resentment for being controlled. It is not so much being protective that is the problem here, it is being 'overprotective'. When carers find that everything in life is centred around the person with the illness to the exclusion of almost everything else then it's probably worth looking at whether this is still the best way of responding. The challenge is when this type of caring leads to family members doing things for others that in the long run they would be better doing for themselves. This way of responding is also a problem when it prevents the carer from moving on with their own life.

An example of 'persecuting' is when family members become aloof, detached, confrontational, critical or underinvolved. The carer might try and make the person with the illness (or other family members) feel guilty or ashamed enough to want to change or 'get their act together'. Unfortunately, using guilt and shame tends not to bring about long-term change and can often make things worse.

The 'victim' response can be when the carer blames someone else for their woes, in such a way that they feel helpless/powerless and avoid taking personal responsibility to make changes. This is not to suggest that the carer reacting in this way does not have genuine suffering – far from it. In fact, the suffering will often be compounded by the stigma associated with mental illness, a poor response from the mental health system, or the lack of appropriate support from family or friends. Unfortunately the suffering, distress and helplessness that family members often feel are likely to continue for themselves and the person with the illness if their reaction roles become rigid.

Changing these patterns can be difficult, particularly if the person has been in a caring role for many years. However, the risk of continuing such patterns is that the person with mental illness may come to view themselves as always being 'unwell', 'disabled' or 'incapable'. This risks the possibility of them losing motivation and feeling helpless and hopeless.

Families need to find a way to care for and help their loved one that also maintains and strengthens relationships, as well as gently supports them on their recovery journey. It is important to find a balance that neither disempowers the person with the illness nor supports a pattern of behaviour that may get in the way of them living their life to the fullest. The same can be said about supporting carers.

Collaboration and relational empowerment

It is clear from both qualitative and quantitative research that families typically want to be involved in clinical decisions. Although recovery is an individual journey, it occurs within an interpersonal context. Therefore, facilitating effective collaboration between the person with the illness and their support network, and between health professionals and family and carers is a critical part of recovery support for the person with the illness and the family. Disempowerment at times appears contagious, so if families and carers feel disempowered it is likely to be reflected in their interactions with the person with the illness. However, empowerment begets empowerment, so if families and carers feel empowered in their interactions with health professions they will be more likely to pass this experience on to the person with the illness. The following areas have been identified as priorities for collaboration.

- Early intervention
- Crisis response
- Treatment plans
- Discharge plans

Early intervention

Families often believe that they become aware of warning signs for relapse before mental health practitioners do. It would not be surprising if this was the case as they typically have more intimate knowledge of the person and more frequent contact. They are therefore likely to notice when something seems different. However, a common complaint is that practitioners are uninterested or unresponsive when family members point to early warning signs. If a relapse does eventuate, the family understandably feels aggrieved.

Crisis response

A crisis is a subjective experience. It is also an intensely stressful experience. Families often report inadequate response to crisis. This is especially the case when the family member with the mental health problem is assessed in a hospital emergency department or by a crisis assessment team and a decision is made to send the person home. Crisis may be as much about the family not coping as the client not coping. An acute admission provides some respite and relief. Returning the client home means there is no relief for the family except perhaps that the client is not as desperately unwell as seemed to be the case. Crisis assessment typically focuses on the mental state of the client with the needs of the family being ignored or at best a minor consideration. Even when family needs are acknowledged, there is rarely effective intervention to assist families.

Treatment plans

Family members are rarely party to treatment plans. Treatment plans are typically developed by the treatment team, often with some consultation with the client. Families may get an overview at a family meeting but rarely receive a copy of the written plan and rarely actively contribute to the development of the plan. On the other hand, practitioners typically expect family members to support the plan or to play a delimited role in implementation of the plan. The research suggests that many families want a much more active role and in some cases would like to be part of the treatment team.

Discharge plans

Failure to consult with families in relation to discharge planning is one of the most contentious issues, especially when discharge is from an acute hospital admission. It is not uncommon for families to report that they first knew their son or daughter had been discharged when he or she turned up at the door. Failure to consult over discharge often feels like betrayal. It also has practical implications. The hospital may believe a person is going home into the care of the family but the family may not be in a position to provide this care at the time of discharge, even if willing to take on the responsibility at some point. At a minimum, families and carers would benefit from consultation regarding the relapse signature of the person with the illness, and what family and carers need to effectively support this person.

What are the barriers to collaboration?

Practitioners typically identify the following as reasons why they fail to collaborate with families.

- Concerns about confidentiality
- Respect for the autonomy of the client

- Difficulty contacting families
- Lack of time
- 'Difficult' families

There is some validity to all of these barriers but much comes down to priority. Working with families is time consuming and even more so when families are 'difficult'. Some clients are ambivalent or even negative about collaboration with families and this means careful negotiation with both parties. Respecting the needs of the family without infantilising the client can be challenging but is very important. While time consuming in the short term, effective collaboration with families may well be cost effective in the longer term, especially if it leads to fewer acute episodes and less need for hospitalisation. Much of the relational 'difficulty' in families is because of the reaction role patterns mentioned above.

The challenge of confidentiality

Practitioners are bound to treat client information as confidential. This means that practitioners cannot share information about a client's mental health or treatment with a family member without the permission of the client. Often clients freely grant permission but it is not unusual for clients to express reservation about sharing information with family members. In these circumstances the negotiation skills of the practitioner are central to a satisfactory outcome.

The following are useful tips when negotiating with a client about disclosing information to family members.

- Explain why family members want or need information.
- Ask the client about specific concerns they have about family members receiving specific information.
- Identify any specific family members the client is or is not happy for the service to communicate with.
- Encourage the client to identify specific things they do not want the family to know and give undertakings in relation to these specifics.
- Write down a list of the information that can be shared with family members that the client can sign and that can be stored in the client record as a reference point for other members of the treating team.
- Make sure everyone in the treating team knows that the client does not want open communication with family members and has a clear understanding of which family members the client has agreed to include in communication with the team and what kinds of information can be shared with these people.
- Don't assume that consent or otherwise is static; check in with the client on a regular basis to determine how they feel about communication with family members.

Problem solving

There is an established evidence base for the effectiveness of a problem-solving framework when working with families. This section will focus on why it is helpful for families and on particular strategies for using problem solving with families.

Aside from psychoeducation and collaboration, the main goal when working with families is helping them to manage the various practical and emotional challenges associated with caring for a person with a mental illness. The evidence suggests that the better family members are able to cope with these challenges, the less stressful the home environment and less need for acute psychiatric care. In turn, fewer acute episodes mean less stress at home and lower burden of care. Having skills to manage stress and to cope with illness is a critical early stage in the personal and relational empowerment journey of the carer.

Problem solving is a therapy approach that facilitates family-generated solutions to problems. It does not mean that the practitioner provides the solutions. Family-generated solutions are likely to be more relevant and more successful because family members know more about their needs and environment than any practitioner can. Family-generated solutions are also empowering and build confidence among family members in their capacity to find solutions.

The role of the practitioner is to help the family clarify the problem and to find novel and practical solutions.

While problem solving seems like a very simple approach to working with people, there are some important things to bear in mind.

- Clarification of the problem should be done carefully – the problem might not be what it seems to be at first glance.
- Avoid the temptation to jump in and offer solutions – often the most workable solutions are those that are either generated by family members or have high levels of family endorsement.
- Practitioner-generated solutions might be most useful when offered as questions, e.g. 'what would happen if …?'.
- When solutions don't work, don't worry – just get back to work with the family.

Strengths

Helping carers to identify and build strength within themselves and their families can assist in terms of finding stability throughout their recovery journeys. However, carers may struggle to identify strengths, things that are going well, and things they can draw strength from. This is particularly difficult when the focus has been on the difficulties, stress and traumas that living with mental illness can bring.

Strengths are all those things that help carers deal with challenges. They are the things that make and keep them strong, reminders of what they are capable of doing and being. Strengths might be some of the attitudes and values carers hold and can include skills and abilities. They can also be external things and people that help carers keep strong. They can be talents, resources, skills and memories that can be draw upon to get through challenging situations. The other way of thinking about strengths is that they help build resilience. Resilience is the ability to handle difficulties and the 'ups and downs' of life without being overcome by them.

It is important to remember that strengths can be developed or expanded upon by setting and working towards goals and turning these goals into actions. So if a carer doesn't feel strong in a particular area that does not mean that this will always be the case. Drawing on existing strengths can help build new strengths.

When the focus is turned to the strengths that different family members have, it can give them a break from focusing on what is 'wrong' or 'lacking' in each other. It can open them up to the possibilities – the *potential* of each individual and the family as a whole. This may lead to carers feeling more hopeful about the future. Also, if carers are looking for the potential and possibilities in others and themselves, they are less likely to get locked into unhelpful roles and reaction patterns.

See Chapter 7 for further strategies to work on building strength.

Peer support

Families often benefit from contact with other people in a similar position. The major benefits of contacts with peers are:

- reassurance through discovering that other people are struggling with similar difficulties
- reassurance through discovering that mental illness affects other ordinary people
- learning how to manage through sharing stories and experiences
- learning from strategies or approaches that other families have found successful
- discovering information or resources that other families know about
- developing contacts and networks that provide new opportunities for the person with mental illness or other family members
- understanding that carers and families can work on their own recovery journeys, and that this is not about abandoning responsibility but rather taking responsibility for the things they can change
- understanding the value of and pathways to taking back their own lives.

Often carers don't think enough about the resources within their community that could be used for support, and stigma will often stop them from reaching out for support, even from people who have had similar experiences to themselves. Peer support can be facilitated and resourced by a clinical or rehabilitation service or can be independent of professional services. Some countries have flourishing carer organisations that offer a wide range of peer-to-peer services and supports. Examples of these are:

- National Alliance on Mental Illness (NAMI) in the US: www.nami.org
- Mental Illness Fellowship of Australia (MIFA): www.mifa.org.au
- Arafmi Australia: http://www.arafmiaustralia.asn.au/recovery.html

The above organisations provide peer-run psychoeducational programmes for families and carers of people with mental illness. The NAMI course is called Family-to-Family and has the following contents.

- Current information about schizophrenia, major depression, bipolar disorder (manic depression), panic disorder, obsessive-compulsive disorder, borderline personality disorder, and co-occurring brain disorders and addictive disorders

- Up-to-date information about medications, side-effects and strategies for medication adherence
- Current research related to the biology of brain disorders and the evidence-based, most effective treatments to promote recovery
- Gaining empathy by understanding the subjective, lived experience of a person with mental illness
- Learning in special workshops for problem solving, listening and communication techniques
- Acquiring strategies for handling crises and relapse
- Focusing on care for the caregiver: coping with worry, stress and emotional overload
- Guidance on locating appropriate supports and services within the community
- Information on advocacy initiatives designed to improve and expand services

(From the NAMI website at http://www.nami.org/Template.cfm?Section=Family-to-Family& lstid=605)

The Australian course is broadly similar and, according to the website covers the following:

- practical information about mental illnesses
- information about the mental health and legal system
- practical frameworks to support people to manage the impact of mental illness on their lives.

Sam's mother is concerned that he is hard to get out of bed in the morning. She tries to rouse him and he just mumbles and turns over and goes back to sleep. It seems worse after his medication increases. Sam says he wants to get some work but she has no idea how he will ever get a job when he is often not up before midday.
   Problem clarification reveals several dimensions to this problem.

- She hates nagging Sam.
- She worries about his future.
- Sam's sleep pattern is causing some conflict between her and Sam's father who thinks she is too soft with him, whereas she thinks it is probably because of the medication and not really Sam's fault.

When brainstorming, Sam's mother comes up with the following.

- Talk with Sam's doctor about his medications.
- Tip a bucket of cold water on Sam at 7am.
- Hand over responsibility to his father for getting him up.
- Stop worrying and just accept that his mental illness means he will never have a normal sleep pattern.
- Check in with Sam about his sleep pattern and work.

When reflecting on strengths, Sam's mother draws strength from the following.

- Sam's doctor seemed genuinely interested and helpful.
- Even though her husband thinks she is too soft with Sam, she knows they will support each other no matter what.
- She knows the personal stories of carers on the Arafmi website have previously given her hope, and that a carer support group is available only 30 minutes drive from her home.
- Her spiritual beliefs.
- The peace she finds in her garden.
- The values of compassion and determination she has.
- Her love for Sam.

After thinking through these possibilities and gathering strength from being in touch with her strengths, she decides she could talk with Sam rather than nagging him and she would like to start with the last of these options. She tries out a few strategies for discussing Sam's sleep pattern with the practitioner. When the opportunity arises, she talks with Sam about his sleep pattern. Sam says he likes the night-time because he feels calmer and less hassled. He does not feel like going to bed before 3am. He does not think the increased medication is making him more drowsy and he is feeling less stressed with the new dose. He has been thinking about work and wondering about some night-shift cleaning. She is very reassured after this conversation and decides the next step is to discuss his situation with her husband, whose business employs cleaning contractors.

Summary

It is important for practitioners to support families and carers with a family member or friend affected by severe mental illness. Recognising the burden of care, immediate educational and stability needs, and readiness to receive support is the first step. At a practical level, families and carers will usually require information about the illness (including causes, trajectory and recovery) and medication, problem-solving and coping strategies, and clarification of available treatments as well as supports for themselves, including peer support options. It is also important to explore existing strengths to assist families to manage challenges associated with care, as well as orienting them towards their own personal and relational empowerment.

References

Barrowclough C, Ward J, Wearden A, Gregg L (2005) Expressed emotion and attributions in relatives of schizophrenis patients with and without substance misuse. *Social Psychiatry and Psychiatric Epidemiology* **40**, 884–91.

Briggs H, Fisher D (2000) *Warning: Caring is a Health Hazard*. Carers Association of Australia: Canberra.

Brown S, Lewis V (1999) *The Alcoholic Family in Recovery: A Developmental Model*. Guilford Press: New York.

Buckley-Walker K, Crowe T, Caputi P (2010) Exploring identity within the recovery process of people with chronic mental illness. *Psychiatric Rehabilition Journal* **33**(3), 219–27.

Butler R, Bauld L (2005) The parents' experience: coping with drug use in the family. *Drugs: Education, Prevention and Policy* **12**(1), 35–45.

Choy A (1990) The winner's triangle. *Transactional Analysis Journal* **20**(1), 40–6.

Clark RE (2001) Family support and substance use outcomes for persons with mental illness and substance use disorders. *Schizophrenia Bulletin* **27**(1), 93–101.

Cummins RA, Hughes J, Tomyn A, Gibson A, Woerner J, Lai L (2007) *The Wellbeing of Australians – Carer Health and Wellbeing*. Australian Centre on Quality of Life: Melbourne, Victoria.

Fulkerson M (2003) Integrating the Karpman drama triangle with choice theory and reality therapy. *International Journal of Reality Therapy* **23**(1), 12–14.

Glynn SM, Cohen AN, Dixon LB, Niv N (2006) The potential impact of the recovery movement on family interventions for schizophrenia: opportunities and obstacles. *Schizophrenia Bulletin* **32**(3), 451–63.

Karp DA, Tanarugsachock V (2000) Mental illness, caregiving, and emotion management. *Qualitative Health Research* **10**(1), 6–25.

Karpman SB (1968) Fairy tales and script drama analysis. *Transactional Analysis Bulletin* **7**(26), 39–43.

Kirby KC, Marlowe DB, Festinger DS, Garvey KA, LaMonaca V (1999) Community reinforcement training for family and significant othes of drug abusers: a unilateral intervention to increase treatment entry of drug users. *Drug and Alcohol Dependence* **56**, 85–96.

McFarlane W (2004) *Multifamily Groups in the Treatment of Severe Psychiatric Disorder*. Guilford Press: New York.

Milliken PJ, Nortcott HC (2003) Redefining parental identity: caregiving and schizophrenia. *Qualitative Health Research* **13**, 100–10.

Moore BC (2005) Empirically supported family and peer interventions for dual diagnosis. *Research on Social Work Practice* **15**(4), 231–45.

Muhlbauer SA (2002) Navigating the storm of mental illness: phases in the family's journey. *Qualitative Health Research* **12**(8), 1076–92.

Needle R, Su S, Doherty W, Laveey Y, Brown P (1988) Familial, interpersonal, and intrapersonal correlates of drug use: a longitudinal comparison of adolescents in treatment, drug-using adolescents not in treatment, and non-drug-using adolescents. *International Journal of Addictions* **23**(12), 1211–40.

Pagnini D (2005) *Carer Life Course Framework: An Evidence-Based Approach to Effective Carer Education and Support*. Carers NSW, Carers Mental Health Professionals: Sydney, Australia.

Ranganathan S (2004) Families in transition: victims of alcoholism and new challenges ahead. *International Journal for the Advancement of Counselling* **26**(4), 399–405.

Rose L, Mallinson RK, Walton-Moss B (2002) A grounded theory of families responding to mental illness. *Western Journal of Nursing Research* **24**, 516–36.

Schlesinger SE, Horberg LK (1994) The "Taking Charge" model of recovery for addictive families. In: Lewis JA (ed) *Addictions: Concepts and Strategies for Treatment*. Aspen Publishers: Gaithersburg, Maryland, pp.233–51.

Schofield N, Quinn J, Haddock G, Barrowclough C (2001) Schizophrenia and substance misuse problems: a comparison between patients with and without significant carer contact. *Social Psychiatry and Psychiatric Epidemiology* **36**, 523–8.

Slade M, Amering M, Oades L (2008) Recovery: an international perspective. *Epidemiologia e Psichiatria Sociale* **17**(2), 128–37.

Chapter 16

Self-Help: Bibliotherapy and Internet Resources

Frank P. Deane and David J. Kavanagh

> Sam is now working and he feels that he no longer needs to be regularly engaged with rehabilitation services. His GP prescribes his medication and Sam knows that he can turn to her if he is in real difficulty. He is, however, aware that he remains susceptible to difficulties – especially symptoms of depression and anxiety and the temptation to drink too much when he is under stress. He would like to be able to access some kind of support or assistance without having to be a regular client of a mental health service.

There is a huge range of self-help resources available to support people to achieve better mental health. Perhaps the best known and most common are self-help books. However, self-help resources include autobiographies, movies, self-help support groups (e.g. AA) and internet materials ranging from information through to cognitive-behavioural therapy (CBT) treatment programmes. The problem with having so many possible self-help resources for a practitioner supporting people in recovery is deciding which to recommend. There are literally tens of thousands of books in the self-help arena and it is estimated that thousands of new self-help books are published each year.

The aim of this chapter is to help mental health workers support people with mental illness through the use of self-help resources. The focus of this chapter is on the use of books (bibliotherapy) and internet self-help programmes with demonstrated effectiveness.

There are several broad steps in the process of supporting people in their use of self-help materials.

1. Clarifying the specific need and context for self-help
2. Identifying appropriate self-help resources
3. Supporting the person in accessing and using the resources
4. Evaluating the effectiveness of the self-help programme

Step 1: Clarify the need for and context of self-help

The advantages of bibliotherapy and internet self-help are that the person can complete them in their own home without necessarily incurring the costs associated with seeing a

Manual of Psychosocial Rehabilitation, First Edition. Edited by Robert King, Chris Lloyd, Tom Meehan, Frank P. Deane and David J. Kavanagh.
© 2012 Blackwell Publishing Ltd. Published 2012 by Blackwell Publishing Ltd.

professional in terms of time and fees. Individuals living in rural areas can have particular difficulty in accessing appropriate care (Griffiths & Christensen, 2007). Others prefer self-help over professional help due to the stigma associated with professional mental health help seeking. There are many reasons why individuals may prefer and seek self-help approaches to their problems.

Understanding when to use a self-help resource depends on the problems the individual is experiencing and the target for change (e.g. knowledge, attitudes, symptoms), the available research evidence supporting their use (to be covered in more detail in the section below) and broader environmental and treatment context issues (stepped care, adjunct to current treatment or access to the internet, etc.). There are some problem domains where self-help programmes have more evidence than others (e.g. bibliotherapy for depression and anxiety; Den Boer et al., 2004).

In what domain does the person need help?

The initial consideration is the domain in which the person needs help and whether there is likely to be an appropriately effective resource. Try to clearly identify the problem domain and likely target. Domains for which there is some research support are listed below in the sections on 'Professional and Expert Consensus' and 'Effectiveness'. Likely targets broadly refer to improvements in knowledge, attitudes (such as reductions in perceived stigma), behaviours (increasing exercise or decreasing sugar intake) or more traditional reductions in symptom severity. Some interventions in specific problem domains (e.g. internet treatment of depression) have more reliable effects in some target outcome areas (e.g. knowledge).

Assess the client's prior self-help experiences

Norcross (2006) makes a number of recommendations for integrating self-help into therapy. One is to assess the clients' prior self-help experiences. This will help clarify those things clients have found previously helpful, whether they can understand and adhere to the tasks and what has changed since their last use of self-help. Changes since last attempts will help focus goals for future self-help material.

Be familiar with the self-help resources and tailor selection

Almost all evidence-based self-help bibliotherapy has involved some level of brief support from a therapist or trained paraprofessional. The amount of support is dependent on how difficult the material is and this highlights the need for clinicians to have at least some familiarity with the self-help material before recommending it.

This familiarity also increases the potential to tailor the selection of material taking into account the individual needs of the person (Norcross, 2006). Part of this tailoring process depends on contextual issues around the use of self-help. For example, increasingly self-help is being recommended as part of what is termed 'stepped care'.

Context of treatment delivery

Stepped care broadly involves providing the 'least restrictive' care available that is likely to produce significant health gains. The term 'least restrictive' in this context usually refers to the lowest impact on patients with regard to cost and inconvenience, but also the minimum amount of treatment provider (therapist) time (Bower & Gilbody, 2005; Salloum, 2010; Tolin *et al.*, 2011). A stepped care model would encourage the use of self-help approaches as first-line treatment before stepping up care to more intensive treatments if improvement does not occur.

It has been suggested that self-help resources might be used while someone is on a waiting list to be seen for professional services. It has been argued that potentially, some individuals will improve and those that don't may be more motivated for face-to-face treatment with a professional (Norcross, 2006). However, a trial of guided self-help for a group of 114 patients awaiting psychological therapy for depression and anxiety failed to find any additional benefit compared to patients who were on the waiting list and received no self-help intervention (Mead *et al.*, 2005). Patients were satisfied with the intervention and whether that provides additional motivation or benefits when receiving professional services is yet to be determined.

Self-help might be used as a supplement when the main focus of face-to-face treatment is on other problem areas or disorder-specific needs. Campbell and Smith (2003) distinguish between bibliotherapy for clinical use versus support/informational use. Clinical use refers to using bibliotherapy with a focus on a clinical condition such as depression. In this circumstance bibliotherapy is often integrated with face-to-face treatment and is usually more closely monitored during these sessions. When bibliotherapy is used for more support or informational purposes the target is not central to the clinical condition – for example, parenting or dealing with chronic illness of a loved one.

The focus of this chapter is more on the clinical use of bibliotherapy. Part of this process involves identifying appropriate evidence-based self-help resources and monitoring treatment response to determine whether further, more intensive treatment is needed in the future.

Step 2: Identifying appropriate self-help resources

There are two primary methods for identifying appropriate self-help resources. The first and preferable method involves consideration of empirical research on their effectiveness. The second occurs when research is not available for particular resources and this relies on professional consensus, usually as a result of surveys of practising mental health professionals or experts.

Effectiveness studies

A broad review of 38 self-help interventions for depression has been undertaken and highlights the wide range of self-help interventions for some mental health problems but found evidence of efficacy for less than a third (Morgan & Jorm, 2008). Examples of interventions with some efficacy included bibliotherapy, computerised interventions, distraction, relaxation training, exercise and pleasant activities. Many of these interventions form components of self-help contained in multicomponent bibliotherapy approaches.

Effectiveness studies have found many biblotherapy treatments helpful for a range of problems including depression (Gregory *et al.*, 2004; Morgan & Jorm, 2008), anxiety (Van Boeijen *et al.*, 2005), alcohol problems (Apodaca & Miller, 2003) and sexual dysfunctions (Van Lankveld, 1998). The mean effect size of bibliotherapy self-help for anxiety and/or depressive disorders in randomised controlled trials is considered moderate to large when compared to placebo or no treatment control groups (e.g. Cuijpers, 1997; Den Boer *et al.*, 2004). Bibliotherapy may be as effective as professional treatment of relatively short duration (Den Boer *et al.*, 2004).

In other problem areas there are promising findings, but more research is needed to strengthen statements of effectiveness (e.g. hypochondriasis: Buwalda & Bouman, 2009; panic disorder: Nordin *et al.*, 2010; tinnitus-related distress: Malouff *et al.*, 2010; parenting: Forehand *et al.*, 2010).

Unfortunately, not all of the effective books or written materials that were used in this research are readily available and access to 'self-help manuals' may be difficult. However, many of the books recommended by professional or expert consensus can be purchased through book stores and many of these also have some degree of research evidence.

Professional and expert consensus

Some guides offer help in the process of selecting appropriate self-help materials, such as the *Authoritative Guide to Self-Help Resources in Mental Health* (Norcross *et al.*, 2000). This guide is based on the results of five national studies in the USA involving surveys of clinical and counselling psychologists. More than 2500 psychologists contributed by rating self-help resources in 28 categories (e.g. anger, anxiety, schizophrenia) on a five-point scale from 'Extremely good' to 'Extremely bad'. The result is a listing of recommendations using a five-star rating system for a wide range of self-help resources including self-help books (bibliotherapy), autobiographies, movies, internet resources and self-help/support groups. The surveys have not been updated since the 1990s when these data were collected. Still, many of these books are likely to be readily available.

Below are the 10 top-rated self-help books related to mental health problems from Norcross *et al.* (2000).

1. *Skills Training Manual for Treating Borderline Personality Disorder* (Linehan M)
2. *Becoming Orgasmic* (Heiman J & LoPiccolo J)
3. *Why Marriages Succeed or Fail* (Gottman J)
4. *The Anxiety and Phobia Workbook* (Bourne E)
5. *Your Defiant Child* (Barkley R & Benton C)
6. *The 36-Hour Day* (Mace N. & Rabins P) (Alzheimer's disease)
7. *The Courage to Heal* (Bass E & Davis L) (abuse and recovery)
8. *Mastery of Your Anxiety and Panic III* (Craske M & Barlow D)
9. *The Relaxation and Stress Reduction Workbook* (Davis M *et al.*)
10. *Feeling Good* (Burns D) (depression)

A more recent review by Redding *et al.* (2008) involved first identifying the 50 best-selling self-help books and then having four experts rate the quality of the books using a standard quality rating scale (e.g. usefulness and consistency with psychological research). Below are the top 10 books along with their quality rating out of 100 (Redding *et al.*, 2008, p.540).

1. *The OCD Workbook* (Hyman BM, 1999) (94)
2. *Dying of Embarrassment* (Markway B, 1992) (92)
3. *The Shyness and Social Anxiety Workbook* (Antony MM, 2000) (92)
4. *Overcoming Compulsive Hoarding* (Neziroglu F, 2004) (90)
5. *Stop Obsessing* (Foa EB, 2001) (90)
6. *The Cyclothymia Workbook* (Prentiss P, 2004) (88)
7. *Bipolar Disorder Demystified* (Castle LR, 2003) (84)
8. *Feeling Good* (Burns DD, 2000) (83)
9. *Overcoming Compulsive Checking* (Hyman BM, 2004) (82)
10. *Obsessive-Compulsive Disorders* (Penzel F, 2000) (81)

There are five self-help books that are present in both the Norcross *et al.* (2000) top-rated list and the top 50 described by Redding *et al.* (2008).

- *Feeling Good* (Burns, 2000)
- *Mind Over Mood* (Greenberger & Padesky, 1995)
- *The Anxiety and Phobia Workbook* (Bourne, 2000)
- *The Relaxation and Stress Reduction Workbook* (Davis, 1995)
- *Trauma and Recovery* (Herman, 1997)

It is notable that these are in the domains of depression and anxiety where there appears to be the most evidence for the effectiveness of bibliotherapy. Probably the most widely used and empirically support book on depression is *Feeling Good* by (Burns, 1999). This is arguably one of the best known and highly supported books by therapists (e.g. Cook *et al.*, 2009; Norcross *et al.*, 2000). Another frequently used book in research trials of bibliotherapy is *Control Your Depression* (Lewinsohn *et al.*, 1986).

For problems associated with recurrent binge eating, there is 'promising' evidence supporting the use of self-help books (Stefano *et al.*, 2006). The books most frequently used and likely to be most readily available are:

- *Overcoming Binge Eating* (Fairburn CG, 1995)
- *Bulimia Nervosa: A Guide to Recovery* (Cooper P, 1993)
- *Getting Better Bit(e) by Bit(e)* (Schmidt UH & Treasure JL, 1993).

The BluePages website (http://bluepages.anu.edu.au/home/) provides an excellent review of depression treatments including bibliotherapy. The rating system is easy to follow and based on reviews of available scientific evidence (e.g. highest rating of three smiley faces means 'These treatments are very useful. They are strongly supported as effective by scientific evidence'). Bibliotherapy receives a rating indicating, 'These treatments are useful. They are supported by scientific evidence as effective, but the evidence is not as strong'. The advantage of this website is that it is periodically updated and provides more recent, user-friendly updates on the effectiveness of various treatments, not only self-help approaches. Further, it provides a list of recommended books (http://bluepages. anu.edu.au/help_and_resources/resources/books/).

Step 3: Supporting the person to use the resources

Typically patients receive some initial instruction and orientation to the self-help materials in a face-to-face meeting. The orientation may include clarifying the goals of completing bibliotherapy in the context of concurrent face-to-face treatment (adjunct). They then take the materials home and work their way through them with brief (5–15 minute) weekly telephone contact from the therapist to check on progress and provide support. The amount and frequency of support provided to maximise effectiveness have not yet been clearly established, but for bibliotherapy at least some telephone contact appears necessary. Generally, the telephone contact involves checking on where the person is up to in their reading, clarifying what they took away from the reading (and associated exercises), any problems they may have in understanding what is being conveyed, any problems in completing exercises, brief advice about how to proceed, encouragement and praise for progress. These contacts are also used to monitor progress with regard to the target goals of bibliotherapy.

Step 4: Evaluating the effects of bibliotherapy

Having clear goals for bibliotherapy that are explicit for the patient usually helps in assessing the effectiveness of bibliotherapy. Clear goals provide clear targets for change that can be monitored over time. The level of evaluation can range from qualitative and informal to involving standardised measures with established reliability and validity that are administered on multiple occasions over time. For example, if the goal is to provide self-help for mild-to-moderate depression, then a depression symptom distress measure might be administered at the start, periodically during treatment and at the end of bibliotherapy. If the goal is to increase motivation or to provide information, less formal assessment of the effects may be possible through the interview process. The main consideration is to get enough information about the effects of bibliotherapy to help the individual make a decision about what, if anything, is needed to address their ongoing needs.

Internet self-help

Internet self-help takes a wide range of forms. For example, in some cases it is essentially bibliotherapy but delivered via the internet. Alternatively, it can be more interactive with the use of video, the potential to customise responses based on client assessment, the provision of supportive blogs, moderated discussion or support groups, or email. As with bibliotherapy, many internet programmes require some level of therapist support, be it through telephone or email contact. It is also advisable for a therapist to be familiar with the content of a website before recommending it to a client. Most of the recommendations regarding administration of bibliotherapy are also applicable to internet self-help, including the need to determine the effectiveness of various resources.

Effectiveness

The empirical research supporting the effects of internet self-help programmes is not as advanced as for bibliotherapy using written materials. However, there are sufficient data to recommend internet-based self-help in several areas such as depression (Morgan & Jorm, 2008) and anxiety. There is growing evidence for some additional disorders such as obsessive-compulsive disorder (Mataix-Cols & Marks, 2006), social phobia (Carlbring *et al.*, 2006) and panic disorder (Carlbring *et al.*, 2006).

New studies describing the effectiveness of web-based applications appear regularly. A good place to get an indication of the effectiveness of new internet self-help applications is at Beacon (www.beacon.anu.edu.au/). This website provides reviews and links to a wide range of online applications for mental health and physical health, for example, alcohol dependence, bipolar disorder, depression, eating distress (body image, anorexia, bulimia), epilepsy, stress, tinnitus, weight and obesity, phobias, post-traumatic stress disorder, resilience, social anxiety, generalised anxiety disorder, obsessive compulsive disorder, pain and panic disorder.

As with the Bluepages site noted above, Beacon provides reviews and ratings by an independent panel of health experts. The reviews include a brief description of the programme, details such as format, target problems, target population (e.g. alcohol), assistance method (e.g. motivational interviewing), length, type of support and primary language. Information about how to access the programme and whether there are fees is also noted. Perhaps most importantly, research evidence for the application is provided. However, there are many more applications than there are programmes with 'good evidence from well-conducted studies'. For example, of the 35 sites reviewed under the category 'Depression', only three had good evidence from well-conducted studies. This is consistent with other published reviews. Griffiths and Christensen (2006) found that only one of three trials for internet treatment of depression had positive results including reductions in depressive symptoms. This effective trial used the MoodGYM web-based programme which is based on cognitive-behavioural therapy (Christensen *et al.*, 2004).

The following are those problem domains and associated sites which have been rated as having good evidence from well-conducted studies from the Beacon site. Unfortunately, not all are currently freely available and able to be used. Some require a subscription and others are closed except for research participant groups. However, we list them here because they may become more freely available as further evidence for their effectiveness accumulates and the need for continuing research trials reduces.

- Alcohol:
  - eCHECKUP TO GO: a prevention program for alcohol use www.echeckuptogo.com
  - Check Your Drinking is a brief online assessment of alcohol use which provides information and some personalised feedback www.checkyourdrinking.net

- Depression:
  - MoodGYM www.moodgym.anu.edu.au (free to use)
  - Virtual Clinic: The Sadness Program www.virtualclinic.org.au
- Eating disorders: Student Bodies targets women at risk of eating disorders http://bml. stanford.edu/multimedia_lab/
- Generalised anxiety: MoodGYM www.moodgym.anu.edu.au (free to use)
- Panic disorder: Panic Online Step 2 (now updated as Panic Stop!) http://www.swinburne. edu.au/lss/swinpsyche/etherapy/programs.html
- Post-traumatic stress disorder: Interapy – PTSD www.interapy.nl
- Social anxiety: Virtual Clinic Shyness program www.virtualclinic.org.au

The Beacon site provides other internet sites and programmes that have less rigorous research evidence but which are still likely to prove helpful for some clients. Given that most of the evidence-based internet interventions have limited access, the reader might like to consider either bibliotherapy or other internet interventions with developing evidence. Among these are the OnTrack programs from the second author of this chapter (www.ontrack.org.au), which include programs on depression, alcohol, support for families and friends, and one on psychosis-like symptoms. Research support for these more recent programs is rapidly growing.

As with bibliotherapy, clinicians recommending internet interventions should be familiar with their content and aware of how they are delivered. Some provide professional support while others are fully automated and provide feedback based on the input of the client.

Summary

There are a large number of self-help resources available to support the treatment of mental health problems. Matching the needs of the client with appropriate forms of self-help is essential. Practitioners should seek out those self-help programmes with the best available research evidence for their effectiveness and need to stay abreast of the rapidly expanding evidence base. This can be accomplished through internet independent review services such as Bluepages and Beacon. Although self-help can be completed without professional support, often a practitioner is needed to help with selection and preparation in relation to self-help programmes. Depending on the self-help resources used, there may also be a need for brief ongoing support and monitoring to assess progress and programme effectiveness.

References

Apodaca TR, Miller WR (2003) A meta-analysis of the effectiveness of bibliotherapy for alcohol problems. *Journal of Clinical Psychology* **59**, 289–304.

Bower P, Gilbody S (2005) Stepped care in psychological therapies: access, effectiveness and efficiency. *British Journal of Psychiatry* **186**, 11–17.

Burns DD (1999) *Feeling Good: The New Mood Therapy*, revised edition. Penguin Putnam: New York.

Buwalda FM, Bouman TK (2009) Cognitive-behavioural bibliotherapy for hypochondriasis: a pilot study. *Behavioural and Cognitive Psychotherapy* **37**, 335–40.

Campbell LF, Smith TP (2003) Integrating self-help books into psychotherapy. *Journal of Clinical Psychology/In Session* **59**, 177–86.

Carlbring P, Furmark T, Steczko J, Ekselius L, Andersson G (2006a) An open ended study of internet-based bibliotherapy with minimal therapist contact via email for social phobia. *Clinical Psychologist* **10**, 30–8.

Carlbring P, Bohman S, Brunt S *et al.* (2006b) Remote treatment of panic disorder: a randomized trial of internet-based cognitive behaviour therapy supplemented with telephone calls. *American Journal of Psychiatry* **163**, 2119–25.

Christensen H, Griffiths K, Jorm A (2004) Delivering interventions for depression by using the internet: randomised controlled trial. *British Medical Journal* **328**, 265.

Cook JM, Biyanova T, Coyne JC (2009) Influential psychotherapy figures, authors, and books: an internet survey of over 2,000 psychotherapists. *Psychotherapy: Theory, Research, Practice, Training* **46**, 42–51.

Cuijpers P (1997) Bibliotherapy in unipolar depression: a meta-analysis. *Journal of Behaviour Therapy and Experimental Psychiatry* **28**, 139–47.

Den Boer PCAM, Wiersma D, van den Bosch RJ (2004) Why is self-help neglected in the treatment of emotional disorders? A meta-analysis. *Psychological Medicine* **34**, 959–71.

Forehand RL, Merchant MJ, Long N, Garai E (2010) An examination of Parenting the Strong-Willed Child as bibliotherapy for parents. *Behavior Modification* **34**, 57–76.

Gregory RJ, Canning SS, Lee TW, Wise JC (2004) Cognitive bibliotherapy for depression: a meta-analysis. *Professional Psychology: Research and Practice* **35**, 275–80.

Griffiths KM, Christensen, H (2006) Review of randomised controlled trials of internet interventions for mental disorders and related conditions. *Clinical Psychologist*, **10**, 16–29.

Griffiths KM, Christensen H (2007) Internet-based mental health programs: a powerful tool in the rural medical kit. *Australian Journal of Rural Health* **15**, 81–7.

Lewinsohn PM, Munoz RF, Youngren MA, Zeiss AM (1986) *Control Your Depression*. Prentice-Hall: New York.

Malouff JM, Noble W, Schutte NS, Bhuller N (2010) The effectiveness of bibliotherapy in alleviating tinnitus-related distress. *Journal of Psychosomatic Research* **68**, 245–51.

Mataix-Cols D, Marks IM (2006) Self-help for obsessive-compulsive disorder: how much therapist contact is necessary? *Clinical Neuropsychiatry: Journal of Treatment Evaluation* **3**, 404–9.

Mead N, MacDonald W, Bower P *et al.* (2005) The clinical effectiveness of guided self-help versus waiting-list control in the management of anxiety and depression: a randomized controlled trial. *Psychological Medicine* **35**, 1633–43.

Morgan AJ, Jorm AF (2008) Self-help interventions for depressive disorders and depressive symptoms: a systematic review. *Annals of General Psychiatry* **7**, 13.

Norcross JC (2006) Integrating self-help into psychotherapy: 16 practical suggestions. *Professional Psychology: Research and Practice* **37**, 683–93.

Norcross JC, Santrock JW, Campbell LF, Smith TP, Sommer R, Zuckerman EL (2000) *Authoritative Guide to Self-Help Resources in Mental Health*. Guilford Press: New York.

Nordin S, Carlbring P, Cuijpers P, Anderson G (2010) Expanding the limits of bibliotherapy for panic disorder: randomized trial of self-help without support but with a clear deadline. *Behavior Therapy* **41**, 267–76.

Redding RE, Herbert JD, Forman EM (2008) Popular self-help books for anxiety, depression, and trauma: how scientifically grounded and useful are they? *Professional Psychology: Research and Practice* **39**, 537–45.

Salloum A (2010) Minimal therapist-assisted cognitive-behavioral therapy interventions in stepped care for childhood anxiety. *Professional Psychology: Research and Practice* **41**, 41–7.

Stefano SC, Bacaltchuk J, Blay SL, Hay P (2006) Self-help treatments for disorders of recurrent binge eating: a systematic review. *Acta Psychiatrica Scandinavica* **113**, 452–9.

Tolin DE, Diefenbach GJ, Gilliam CM (2011) Stepped care versus standard cognitive-behavioral therapy for obsessive-compulsive disorder: a preliminary study of efficacy and costs. *Depression and Anxiety* **28**, 314–23.

Van Boeijen CA, van Balkom AJLM, van Oppen P, Blankensetien N, Cherpahath A, van Dyck R (2005) Efficacy of self-help manuals for anxiety disorders in primary care: a systematic review. *Family Practice* **22**, 192–6.

Van Lankveld JJDM (1998) Bibliotherapy in the treatment of sexual dysfunctions: a meta-analysis. *Journal of Consulting and Clinical Psychology* **66**, 702–8.

Part V
Bringing It All Together

Chapter 17

Reviewing and Clarifying an Individual Rehabilitation Programme

David J. Kavanagh and Robert King

Sam's practitioner has now identified several issues that Sam is facing, and she and Sam have been working on several of them over the last 3 months. They are making progress together, but today Sam said he was feeling frustrated about not achieving more.

Sam's rehabilitation practitioner is struck by how many issues she and Sam have identified, and feels confused about how to proceed. It is time to take stock, prioritise the remaining issues, and revise the rehabilitation programme. She decides to make a summary, and try to see how the issues may relate to each other.

On readministration of the HoNOS (see Chapter 3), Sam's acute symptoms, social withdrawal and problems with self-care have now resolved, and after doing weekly cognitive remediation (see Chapter 9), his concentration and memory are much improved. However, he has some problems getting to sleep (often awake until 2–3am, also often sleeping in the afternoons), motivation, emotional responsiveness and lack of pleasure. There was a question of whether his medication was contributing to his fatigue, lack of energy and restlessness; recent medication reductions he negotiated with his psychiatrist do seem to have reduced these problems (as confirmed by readministration of the LUNSERS (see Chapter 3). He continues to take his medication daily (with occasional lapses), despite being dissatisfied with the side-effects.

As his acute symptoms resolved, insight into his problems and awareness of their impact on his life appeared to worsen his dysphoria. He expressed a lack of confidence in being able to address functional challenges, and this thought (together with his belief that his life was destroyed) appeared to both be exacerbated by dysphoria and to contribute to it continuing. After some weeks with very high levels of distress, his Kessler-6 score has recently been much improved (see Chapter 2), although it remains in the clinical range. Sam says that he found fun activities did make a difference (see Chapter 8) but he found it hard to keep going. In particular, he started practising the guitar again for a time, but he has not touched it now for 4 weeks. Nor has he been very physically active over the last 6 weeks (see Chapter 13).

After a motivational interview (see Chapter 6), Sam attempted to stop smoking. This attempt lasted 5 weeks, ending after an argument with his girlfriend, Angela, over her missing her own medication doses. He went out drinking, and accepted a cigarette from someone at the bar, and is now smoking as much as before.

Sam went to a group session at the centre about his drinking (see Chapter 13) but at the time, his social anxiety was too high to continue. Instead, he did some segments of an internet-based alcohol intervention on one of the centre's computers (see Chapter 16), with occasional help from one of the staff. Apart from the incident when he returned to smoking,

Manual of Psychosocial Rehabilitation, First Edition. Edited by Robert King, Chris Lloyd, Tom Meehan, Frank P. Deane and David J. Kavanagh.

he has only been drinking 1–2 times a week, and has not had more than two drinks (20 g ethanol) on any occasion (see Chapter 2).

Sam completed the centre's group social skills programme (see Chapter 11), including segments on writing a resumé and fielding interview questions: his social performance is now considerably better than when he started at the centre, and he no longer has significant social anxiety. He has even started participating in an online peer support programme one or twice (see Chapter 14).

Sam also completed a programme on transportation (see Chapter 12) and now has no difficulty using public transport. He attended some cooking lessons at the rehabilitation centre, but Angela still does most of the cooking.

He obtained an evening job as a cleaner, and both his mood and sleeping improved. However, he lost the job after a week, when he did not turn up for work on two successive evenings (he said he was tired, after working on Angela's car during the day). Financial worries continue, and he still has some problems managing a budget (see Chapter 12). This remains a source of conflict with Angela.

Sam is now staying overnight at Angela's flat more than he is at home. This has reduced the tension at home to some extent, but Sam's mother still worries about him. She has usually been the first person to notice his episodes emerging, and it is usually she who approaches services for help. Sam becomes irritated by her questioning him about how he is feeling, and says she treats him like a child. Staying with Angela helps him to avoid his mother's questioning.

Despite his achievements, Sam still lacks some optimism and a sense of control over the future on an Empowerment scale (see Chapter 4). Similarly, a readministration of a WHOQOL-BREF (see Chapter 5) shows that scores on psychological health and environmental quality of life remain low.

The complexity of this picture is not unusual. Nor is the fact that progress is patchy and is not always fully sustained. There is a risk that both client and practitioner might focus on what has not been achieved, rather than on positive achievements. Summarising those achievements can make an important contribution to the optimism and self-efficacy of both parties.

A case summary of this kind can also identify inter-relationships between issues, and changes that have (or could have) an impact on multiple important aspects of Sam's life. An example of how this summary can be used is provided below.

Together with Sam, his practitioner makes a list of his achievements since they began working together (Table 17.1).

Sam is amazed to see the list. 'Wow! We have done quite a lot in 3 months, I guess. I hadn't put it together.' However, he still felt frustrated that he hadn't been able to persist with some things. It felt like he had slipped back in many ways.

Sam's practitioner suggests they make a list of things that may still need some attention (Table 17.2, column 2). Then, they review the things that Sam values most – he now see them as satisfaction with life, physical health and better relationships (Table 17.2, last column). They brainstorm some ideas about how they could work on remaining issues (Table 17.2, column 3).

Table 17.1   Sam's list of achievements.

Things I have achieved	What is better
Took medication regularly	No more hallucinations or odd ideas, less unhappy
Came to most rehab sessions and usually tried out ideas between sessions	Some things are getting better
Talked to doctor about medications (he cut the dose)	Less restless and tired
Looked after myself better (washed, shaved every day, wore deodorant, cleaned my teeth, went to the dentist)	Now look/smell better
Quit smoking for 5 weeks (!)	Felt much healthier, more able to breathe when didn't smoke. Fewer arguments with Angela
Did computer training programme for my attention and memory (and remembered to come to most sessions!)	Can concentrate and remember things better now
Went to the social skills group, despite feeling anxious about it. Took part in a couple of online peer support sessions	Less anxious around people, and mixing more. Can now write my CV and do a job interview
Tried to play the guitar and do other fun things, was more active for about 2 weeks	Less unhappy when I did them, felt fitter when I was active
Went to a group session and did some work on a computer for my drinking. Cut down my drinking to 1–2 times a week, no more than two drinks (still doing it!)	A bit more money, feel better the next day
Went to two cooking classes	Could cook a potato, make a hamburger after the classes (not sure I still can)
Finished a transport group	Can catch the bus to the supermarket and the city
Got a cleaning job for a few days	More money that week
Kept seeing Angela, told her I love her, made up after arguments	Relationship with Angela has now lasted 3 months – the longest ever

When faced with many issues, it is often hard to know where to start. We recommend that readers give this question some thought before carrying on to see what Sam's practitioner does. It is likely that different practitioners and clients may come to different conclusions about how to proceed, and there may be many directions that could lead to positive outcomes. It can be helpful to discuss ideas with the rehabilitation team to obtain others' perspectives, and then take some of the discussion points back to the client.

Some considerations that help with this process include the following.

- What is most important to the client? In particular, what links most closely to their core values (see Chapter 7)?
- What is most urgent?
- What is a focus that will be likely to give early gains and build confidence?
- What things may impact on multiple areas, so that widespread gains are obtained?

Table 17.2   Sam's list of things he still wants to work on.

Priority	Things I still want to work on	What I'll do	Things I value
6	Still feel down, future still doesn't look good, still feel I can't do things, still dissatisfied with life	Looking at what I've achieved each month Work on things on this list	➡**Satisfied with life** **Physical health** **Better relationships**
=3	Feeling bored, not having enough fun	Start doing fun activities again, including playing guitar	➡**Satisfied with life** →**Physical health** →**Better relationships**
=3	Feeling unfit	Get back to being active, including walking, playing with Angela's daughter Talk to Angela about what we eat Go back to cooking and diet planning classes next month	➡**Satisfied with life** ➡**Physical health** →**Better relationships**
6	Getting to sleep	Try to stay awake in the afternoon Maybe do an online sleep program with my practitioner next month	→**Satisfied with life** ➡**Physical health** →**Better relationships**
1	Smoking again	Start another quit smoking attempt	➡**Satisfied with life** ➡**Physical health** ➡**Better relationships**
2	No job, not enough money	Go to the employment service for help in my job search	➡**Satisfied with life** →**Physical health** ➡**Better relationships**
5	Mum worrying about me, hassling me	See if she will come for more sessions on schizophrenia, and how she can cope Staying with Angela, having a job and more money will help her feel less worried Learn how to deal with Mum's concern – I love her and like her helping but need to get her to back off a bit	➡**Satisfied with life** **Physical health** ➡**Better relationships**
4	Arguments with Angela	Talk to her about what she wants Help her with parenting tasks Help her deal with her own issues	➡**Satisfied with life** **Physical health** ➡**Better relationships**

Sam and his practitioner link the ideas with Sam's core values (see Table 17.2). They make arrows thicker when relationships are stronger.

The number of arrows coming from an action and the thickness of those arrows give clues on what Sam sees as his priorities.

When Sam and his practitioner look at the table, they notice how important it is to Sam to stop smoking. He thinks this success would give him confidence to address other things in his life as well. It may even help him keep a job – after all, he used to spend a lot of time on smoking breaks when he worked in the past. Stopping smoking may also reduce the arguments with Angela; he now realises that her concern was not just about money, it was about the effect of the smoke on her daughter. Sam now shares this concern; Angela's daughter is becoming an important part of his life and he does not want to harm her in any way.

Sam's practitioner tells him how proud she was that he lasted 5 weeks off cigarettes, and had reduced the dose of nicotine replacement to a low level. This meant that he had come through the worst of the withdrawal and had clearly resisted many temptations to smoke. What they needed to do now was work out how to get started again, and how to resist cigarettes if he becomes upset, as he did after the argument with Angela. Sam agrees, and says that he could maybe call his mother and see if he could visit if he was upset and tempted to smoke. Together, Sam and his practitioner review the main reasons to stop smoking, past successes, social support strategies and ways to resist temptation (see Chapter 6). They make a plan to get started next Monday.

Sam would value a job very highly; it is something, he says, that would make him feel 'normal'. It would reduce some of the stress with Angela; he would like to look after her and her daughter, and help rent a house where she can play (they are currently in a small flat). If he had a job, he thinks his mother would also be less anxious, and his father would put less pressure on him as well. Sam's practitioner calls a local job agency, which makes an appointment for Sam the following week. Sam's practitioner reminds him about the training he did on writing a resumé and answering interview questions, and offers to arrange for him to have some more interview practice over the coming week. Sam seems excited about the idea.

Sam says that both these goals may be easier to achieve if he tries to get fit and have more fun; maybe he could start walking each day or play with Angela 's daughter after school in the park while Angela makes dinner. Sam also says he wants to start playing the guitar again. His practitioner says he may have a lot on in the coming days but that it would be great if he were able to fit that in. She suggests that it may be another strategy he could use when he felt a craving for cigarettes. If he can get a job, he will be able to afford some lessons as well. Sam and his practitioner revise the previous menu of activities he can choose from each day, and plan how he will make sure he does them (see Chapter 8).

Sam is confident he can try these three things over the coming month; he rates his confidence about staying off cigarettes for a month as 60%, going for job interviews as 65% and doing more fun activities as 75% (see Chapter 6).

Sometimes, clients will be enthusiastic to try to address many things at once. It is important to remember that clients often surprise us with their accomplishments. However, we seek to help them maintain a focus on the things they most want to achieve, and to be proud of partial achievement of their goals. We also try to ensure that the multiple goals do not induce stress that leads to symptomatic exacerbations. So, we encourage them to try as much as they feel able to do, while not feeling they have to do them all, or that they have failed if they only meet some goals or achieve only some steps toward their goals.

Sam thinks that these goals will also make a difference to many of the other issues. Both his mother and Angela will be happier if he does these things, and if he is more active during the day, he is less likely to have a daytime nap and is more likely to sleep at night. He won't forget his other priorities, but will delay working on them in earnest while he works on the first three.

This example shows how a careful summary of issues, and their relationship to core values (see Chapter 7), can help both the practitioner and client identify priorities and potential steps to their accomplishment.

The example also reminds us that the rehabilitation process is usually not confined to the one service. Sam's practitioner is not an employment expert. However, she does know a good local job agency. While it does not specialise in special placements, she has a contact there who appreciates the difficulties faced by people with mental disorders who are seeking work after a period of unemployment, and will keep trying even if the first job does not work out. If necessary, she can also help Sam to negotiate social security benefits, locate an agency that may be able to help him find affordable housing, or assist Sam to obtain inexpensive legal advice.

While doing this review, Sam's rehabilitation worker is surprised to notice how much she still does not know.

- She has not seen Angela for some time, to follow up on her medication adherence after the efforts to address that (see Chapter 10). She wonders whether Angela is still experiencing mood swings, how Sam would cope with another manic episode, and whether childcare arrangements during an episode could be less intrusive and destabilising. She remembers that Angela's relationship with her psychiatrist was deteriorating some weeks back – had that improved? Had she discussed a plan with her psychiatrist for early intervention if her own symptoms deteriorate? Is she well enough to help detect early signs of potential relapse for Sam, and help him take action quickly?
- Noting that both Sam and Angela have had similar sleep problems, she wonders how these may relate to each other. Do they keep each other awake? Do they help each other deal with insomnia?
- Similarly, she wonders whether Angela may also have been controlling her drinking, and if strategies are needed for each to maintain control if the other lapses.
- She has never asked about how Angela's daughter and Sam relate to each other, whether Sam takes an active role in her parenting, and about the effects of that relationship on Sam.
- She had forgotten that Angela's former partner is in jail. What will happen when he is released? She notes that domestic violence was an issue in the past.
- Although she has had a session with Sam's mother, she needs to know more about the strengths and areas of conflict in Sam's relationship with his parents, what they know about Sam's disorder, functional aspects of their current attempts to cope with their own distress and support Sam, and ways in which Sam would like them to support his efforts at independence (see Chapter 19).

Despite the practitioner having invested considerable effort in assessment, there remain many questions, particularly around relationships with key people in the client's social network. Detailed assessments of relationships and of the needs of families and friends can be missed by services, as they invest their primary effort in assisting the focal client. However, as we see in the case summary, these relationships may be critical to success, and people around the identified client are likely to be profoundly affected by their disorder.

It is tempting to criticise the practitioner for having missed these aspects, but it is important to recognise that initial assessment is often undertaken under time pressure, and key information may not always be disclosed until there is a strong, trusting relationship with the practitioner. Furthermore, new challenges emerge as the person becomes less symptomatic and more functional.

In fact, formulations are always just guesses, based on the information that is at hand at the time. Assessment is therefore not just something that occurs at the start of rehabilitation. Inquiry and hypothesis testing is a theme that is interwoven throughout the rehabilitation process, informing it and being informed by advances, setbacks and incidental facts that emerge in each session. Periodically, it is important to take stock of these emerging data, as Sam's practitioner has, and see how the new information and changes to the client's circumstances and skills affect the picture of what may need to happen next.

In a later joint interview with Angela, Sam tells her about his plans to seek work and stop smoking. Angela is sceptical but says she will help him in any way she can. He asks her to help him take his mind off his craving when he asks her to. She is happy that he wants to become more involved in parenting, and says it would be really helpful if he could help her care for her daughter in the afternoons.

Angela and Sam are clearly very close. Sam's practitioner asks if they had discussed how they can keep each other well, and whether they had a plan to get help if they were at risk of a relapse. Angela offered to help Sam make his plan with the rehabilitation practitioner, and said she would take Sam when she next went to her own doctor, so they could talk through her own plan. (Note that this idea was not in the list Sam developed in Table 17.2: it was an action that emerged from the joint interview but in retrospect should perhaps have been anticipated from the case summary).

Over the next 3 months, Sam's practitioner also has three sessions with Sam and his parents, using strategies described in Chapter 15. They discuss the disorder and the great strides that Sam is making in his recovery. As Sam thought, his mother is relieved to hear he is trying to get a job and to stop smoking, but remains worried that he may not cope and may become unwell. She is reassured by the plan that Sam and Angela have made, and offered to help. Sam and his practitioner agree that if Sam's mother notices that he seems unwell, she will call his practitioner, who will try to see Sam as soon as possible. Sam's father says very little through the interview, but seems pleased he is seeking a job.

These interviews greatly increase the chance of ultimate success, by increasing social support for Sam's attempts and for his relapse risk, and by reducing some of the stress that those relationships had been causing in the past. More support for Angela and for Sam's parents may be needed in the future, especially if he has a setback or his circumstances change (e.g. if the relationship with Angela ended). However, a start has been made.

Summary

Like many clients, Sam's issues are complex but he has surprising strengths and has made substantial strides, despite his severe disorder. Often, the picture is less positive: clients may have multiple acute episodes and may show a deteriorating course, despite substantial effort to assist their functional recovery. Our work is with brain disorders, which may only partially respond to even the best possible rehabilitation or pharmacotherapy programme.

As we emphasised in Chapter 4, recovery does not necessarily mean an absence of ongoing problems: it is making the most of life and of our resources, not letting our lives be defined by a disorder, retaining meaning, purpose and satisfaction. This vision is not just one for our clients. Without it, we as practitioners will become disheartened and frustrated. It is useful to keep in mind the courage and persistence of particular clients with very severe disorders; the strength and resilience that they and their families display in the face of terrible adversity are an inspiration for us, as we keep trying to help them and their peers to the best of our ability.

Chapter 18

Programme Evaluation and Benchmarking

Tom Meehan, Robert King and David J. Kavanagh

Sam has been referred to a substance misuse programme as his alcohol intake was affecting his functioning (a brief overview of the programme is provided in Chapter 12). While Sam has shown some interest in the programme, he has been asking questions about the benefits of attending. When you last mentioned the programme to him, he enquired 'how can you be sure this programme will help me?' and 'if I stop drinking will the programme help me to stay sober?' You find it difficult to answer these questions as the programme is relatively new and has not been fully evaluated.

Evaluation is an ongoing process of asking questions, reflecting on the answers to these questions and implementing change based on the information received. Evaluation provides a systematic means of learning from experience. Organisations, like individuals, have a capacity for self-deception either through over- or undervaluing their achievements. The evaluation process introduces a dimension of objectivity.

Evaluation is critical at all levels of an organisation. At the macro level, it is necessary to ensure ongoing evaluation of the key policy and strategic directions. At the micro level, evaluation is more likely to be concerned with establishing whether or not a specific programme should be continued, modified or ceased. In the rehabilitation field, evaluation studies are frequently conducted to:

- contribute to decisions about the overall benefits of a programme – which clients tend to benefit from the programme and under what conditions?
- contribute to decisions about programme expansion, continuation, modification or termination – what works/does not work and why?
- obtain evidence to secure support for the programme – demonstrate effectiveness
- gain a better understanding of the processes (structural, financial, etc.) affecting the programme
- ensure that the programme remains responsive to the needs of the target group (to prevent 'upmarket shift' in service delivery, i.e. admits clients who were not intended for the programme)
- ensure programme fidelity – the programme continues to be provided as intended.

Manual of Psychosocial Rehabilitation, First Edition. Edited by Robert King, Chris Lloyd, Tom Meehan, Frank P. Deane and David J. Kavanagh.

In effect, evaluation is concerned with determining whether or not a psychosocial rehabilitation intervention worked as it was supposed to work. Evaluation is strongly linked to quality assurance and generates information we can use to develop or sometimes even abandon programmes or interventions.

Approaches used in evaluating rehabilitation programmes

There are many approaches that can be used to evaluate rehabilitation interventions, each with different terms and language. Some of these employ experimental approaches using treatment and control groups while others use a quality improvement approach (such as collecting data on a single group and making improvements based on those data). It is important to discuss different approaches with service providers and other key players such as consumers prior to deciding on any one approach. It is clear that the approach required to evaluate a given programme will depend on a range of factors which must be considered by the evaluator or evaluation team at the time of evaluation. These are outlined in Table 18.1.

Having addressed the questions outlined in Table 18.1, the evaluator will be in a better position to select an approach to guide the evaluation. While a number of different approaches exist, most are based on the 'structure', 'process', 'outcome' model for assessment of quality of care proposed by Donabedian in his classic paper in 1966. Donabedian's model is based on robust theory underpinning programme evaluation more generally. One approach closely aligned to that of Donabedian is the Context, Input, Process and Product (CIPP) Model developed by Stufflebeam (1971).

Table 18.1   Issues to consider prior to commencing an evaluation.

Factor	Issues to consider
Purpose	What is the purpose of the evaluation? What are the key questions/objectives to be addressed? What do key players (staff, clients, managers, etc.) expect to gain from the evaluation? Are there any other/hidden agendas?
Constraints	What are the constraints on the evaluation? These may include cost, time, expertise, computers, office space, staff, etc.
Target group	Who is the target group: staff, clients, or both? Are there any ethical or industrial factors that would make it difficult to recruit participants?
Budget	How much funding is allocated to the evaluation? Will this be sufficient to address the evaluation objectives?
Key players	Is the co-operation of key individuals required to enable the evaluation to be carried out? Have these been engaged in discussions concerning the evaluation?
Ethical issues	Will ethical clearance be required? How long will approval take?
Reporting	How will reporting of findings be carried out? This may be in the form of a single report at the conclusion of the evaluation or by progress reports throughout the evaluation

The Context, Input, Process and Product Model

The CIPP Model uses a systems approach to evaluation. A basic system requires input, process and output. Stufflebeam added 'context' and relabelled 'outcome' with the term 'product' to achieve the Context, Input, Process and Product (CIPP) approach to evaluation. The basic components of the model are described in Table 18.2.

Context evaluation

This component of the evaluation process examines the context of care provision. The focus here is the goals of service/programme provision. Are these aligned to policy and appropriate for the service? Data collected under this component of the evaluation could include:

- the goals and eligibility criteria for admission to the programme
- characteristics of clients admitted (age, gender, background, level of disability, etc.). Do these meet the eligibility criteria?

In effect, context evaluation explores the question: Are the clients being admitted to the rehabilitation programme the clients whom the program was established to treat?

Input evaluation

Input evaluation requires an examination of the services and interventions provided. It focuses on whether the 'inputs' (e.g. staffing levels, staff qualifications, costs, etc.) are appropriate to meet the objectives and goals of the service (described in the previous section on context evaluation). Data collected under this component of the evaluation could include:

- staffing levels, staffing mix, qualifications and experience
- details of interventions planned for clients
- overall cost of providing service.

The key question to be answered here is: Are the interventions provided capable of meeting the needs of the clients in the programme?

Table 18.2   The CIPP approach to evaluation.

Evaluation	Focus	Key questions considered
Context evaluation	Planning of programme	What are the goals of the programme? Are these based on some assessment of need?
Input evaluation	Structure of programme	How well do the interventions provided meet the needs of clients in the programme?
Process evaluation	Implementation of programme	Is the programme being provided as planned? If not, why not?
Product (outcome) evaluation	Outcomes of programme	Is the programme working? Should it be continued, modified or abandoned?

Process evaluation

This component explores the extent to which planned interventions are actually implemented. In other words, it provides an examination of the interventions provided by different staff groups/members over a given period (e.g. 1 week). The issue here is programme fidelity (whether the programme was delivered in accordance with the programme manual, assuming there is some kind of manual). If the programme was delivered differently, the evaluation seeks to determine the reasons for the variation and what effect, if any, the variation had on the success of the programme. Data collected under this component of the evaluation could include:

- description of the activities provided, work practices, programme fidelity
- drop-out rates (attrition) are considered and the evaluation determines whether this rate is typical for the type of programme and target population. Other indicators of engagement are the average number of programme sessions completed and the proportion of programme tasks completed by participants
- how participants experienced the programme. This may include rating of enjoyment, usefulness and relevance, and impact on self-efficacy (capacity to do the things taught in the programme).

The key question to be answered here is: Are the interventions provided in keeping with those that were planned?

Product (outcome) evaluation

This is the final component of the evaluation process and examines whether the programme achieved the stated goals. For example, a healthy eating programme may aim to change eating habits, so that participants eat more fresh fruit and vegetables, less fat and less salt. Outcome is different from impact or process. A programme participant might find a programme enjoyable and might learn about the food pyramid (process) without changing actual eating behaviour (outcome).

While most rehabilitation programmes have a focus on client outcomes, staff outcomes (such as stress, job satisfaction, perceptions of achievements, team functioning, skills, etc.) can also be explored.

Assessment here is likely to focus on:

- outcomes for clients (which could include length of stay, changes in functioning, reduction in risk, reduction in substance misuse, etc.). In effect, this component of the evaluation will be concerned with determining whether participants acquired new knowledge or developed new skills during the course of the programme and if this has resulted in improved functioning
- outcomes for staff (which could include satisfaction with work, perceptions of team functioning, perceptions of individual performance and achievements, stress, burnout, etc.).

The key question asked here is: How well has the programme achieved its goals?

It is clear that an evaluation may focus on all or some of the components outlined. For example, a rehabilitation team may be more interested in the outcomes of a given programme (rather than the other components) and the evaluator will need to clarify this with the rehabilitation team prior to data collection. Indeed, it is recommended that the rehabilitation team provide terms of reference (ToR) for the evaluation or a written proposal detailing the questions to be addressed. This will ensure that the 'deliverables' from the evaluation will be as expected and address the questions posed by the rehabilitation team.

Evaluation methods

Two broad approaches to evaluation are commonly used: qualitative methods and quantitative methods. Typically evaluations use mixed methods (both qualitative and quantitative).

Qualitative methods may include observation of programme implementation, review of programme documents and interviews with programme participants. Qualitative methods are systematic and are designed to extract themes or make judgements about matters such as programme fidelity. *Quantitative methods* use measurements to assign numerical values to programme impact and outcome. These measurements may take the form of satisfaction surveys, standardised outcome scales (see Section 1 of this book) or measures such as the number of days a person has worked or earnings (if, for example, a programme outcome was participant employment).

A worked example

To illustrate the assessment process we will consider how we might evaluate Sam's substance misuse programme as it is described in Chapter 12.

This is an eight-session group programme. The brief manual set out in Chapter 12 is typical of the kind of manual you might expect to find in a practice setting. It is much less developed than a manual for a research programme: it simply sets out in summary form a week-by-week schedule of activities and tasks. The programme does include some 'built-in' evaluation processes, which will provide a useful starting point, but these will not be sufficient for the more rigorous evaluation we will develop here.

A programme evaluation would not just be done on one person, although evaluating Sam's responses to it may provide indicative data on the potential issues that will arise when more people undertake a similar programme. The same logic can be applied to an individual or a group. However, the worked example below assumes that Sam is one of several clients who have undertaken the programme.

Developing a programme logic

A programme logic is a logical statement that sets out what a programme aims to achieve and identifies the resources and processes necessary to achieve the specified outcomes. It may be represented in the form of a diagram or a flow chart or it may be simply a statement or series of statements. When a programme is simply outlined as in this example, the starting point is to construct the programme logic.

The first step is to identify expected programme outcomes. In this case, the programme outcomes can be inferred from the title and content of the programme and from the kind of people who are referred into the programme. It is clear that the main purpose of the programme is to reduce substance misuse. It would therefore be expected that programme completers would show a reduction in substance misuse.

The second step is to identify programme inputs – the resources necessary to achieve the outcomes. In this case the inputs are one or more group facilitators, a suitable space for a group to meet, an activity schedule and various other resources such as printed exercises, questionnaires, information and resource handouts and completion certificates.

The third step is to set out the theory that explains how participation in the programme leads to the designated outcome. In this case, it is clear that the underlying programme logic is that people will reduce substance misuse when they:

- can manage cravings
- better understand the link between self-esteem and substance misuse
- can use cognitive strategies to overcome low self-esteem
- understand the relationship between stress and substance misuse
- can use problem-solving strategies and relaxation to deal with stresses and difficulties
- understand the relationship between social pressure and substance misuse
- can use assertiveness and other social skills to resist social pressure to use substances
- understand the importance of being able to substitute other enjoyable activities for substance misuse
- have identified and tried out enjoyable activities that are a safe alternative to substance misuse.

There are various psychological theories that sit behind this logic but they are not relevant to programme evaluation. However, programme evaluation may well be interested in the extent to which participants achieve the knowledge and/or skill specified in each of the bullet points above because the programme logic suggests that it is through acquisition of this knowledge and skill that the ultimate outcome of reduction in substance misuse is achieved.

Evaluating implementation of Sam's substance misuse programme

- A thorough evaluation would require the evaluator to observe sessions or review videotapes of sessions to determine whether or not the programme was implemented as described in the manual.
- In some cases, psychosocial rehabilitation programmes have established fidelity scales that provide a checklist approach to recording evaluation of fidelity. For an example, see Teague *et al.* (1998). However, most programmes will not have a fidelity scale, and the evaluator will have to develop a simple tool that enables fidelity to be assessed. Checklists can be used to structure evaluations of videotapes, or they can be used

by practitioners to confirm that they included specific elements in the session and implemented them correctly. The latter use of the scales relies on the practitioner's grasp of the critical elements in the programme, and their ability to observe their own performance accurately.

- A less rigorous evaluation bases determination of fidelity on a structured interview with one or more programme facilitators plus review of any records or chart entries maintained in relation to the programme. The evaluator would note variations or omissions and explore reasons for these. The evaluator would also seek advice from the facilitator as to the expected impact of variations or omissions.

Evaluating engagement in Sam's substance misuse programme

The evaluator will want to know:

- how easy it was to recruit participants into the programme and the pattern of attendance. In particular, the evaluator will want to know the numbers who agreed to participate and completed the programme, the mean number of sessions attended by each participant and the average number of participants in attendance at each session. Where possible, this information should be benchmarked against participation patterns for similar programmes
- the amount and quality of engagement and participation in programme activities, including exercises completed during sessions and homework activities between sessions
- (in a more thorough evaluation) reasons for dropping out of the programme or for missing sessions, obtained via interviews with participants. These interviews can also explore programme impact (see below).

Evaluating the impact/process of the programme on participants

Impact evaluation for a programme such as this is moderately complex.

- In part, it will mean finding out from participants how they experienced the programme. This will often make use of a standard satisfaction survey (see Chapter 5) but may also make use of more open-ended information obtained by means of a semi-structured interview.
- A more in-depth evaluation will explore the experience of each of the major components rather than comprising a global evaluation only. This level of evaluation is especially useful when planning changes to a programme.
- A thorough impact evaluation also requires a determination of the extent to which the programme improved participants' knowledge, self-efficacy and skills. The programme logic provides the framework for identifying the relevant variables. When we developed the programme logic for Sam's programme, we identified nine units of knowledge and skill that a participant might expect to develop as a result of participation in the programme. Ideally, an evaluation will use before-and-after measures to evaluate changes in knowledge and skill in each specified area.

Evaluating programme outcomes

This is the single most important part of any programme evaluation. The purpose of the programme is to achieve outcomes. No matter how good the implementation, programme participation or programme impact, if it does not achieve specified outcomes, it is failing. In this case, Sam and other participants enrolled in the programme to reduce the level of substance misuse. This means that the key outcome evaluation questions will concern changes in severity and frequency of substance misuse over the course of the programme and the extent to which these changes are sustained beyond programme participation. This means that it is important to obtain reliable data about substance misuse at baseline (prior to commencing the programme) and programme completions and at follow-up (3 and 6 months may be realistic). Chapter 2 contains examples of measures that can be used for this purpose.

When interpreting outcome, it is important to have reasonable reference points. Not all participants in a substance misuse programme can be expected to reduce their substance misuse. Reference to relevant outcome literature assists in determining reasonable and expected outcomes. Outcomes in real-world settings are typically somewhat weaker than those in research settings; while we strive for the best outcomes, some allowance needs to be made for the lower resources available to conduct the programme and the greater complexity in client problems that are often experienced in applications to routine practice.

Benchmarking rehabilitation services

The benchmarking of performance indicators is another form of programme evaluation. Although benchmarking has its origins in industry, the process is gaining currency in the mental health field as a means of improving service provision (Meehan *et al.*, 2007). Bullivant (1994) defined benchmarking as an activity concerned with the 'systematic process of searching for and implementing a standard of best practice within an individual service or similar groups of services'. Thus, benchmarking could occur within a single organisation with similar units (internal benchmarking) or between organisations with a similar focus (i.e. rehabilitation of individuals with severe disability) known as 'collaborative' benchmarking. Regardless of scope, having identified high-performing organisations, the task is to identify and emulate the clinical/administrative practices that lead to superior performance (Berg *et al.*, 2005).

In practice, participating organisations agree to share information about their performance on a number of key domains such as efficiency, effectiveness and safety. The collection and reporting of performance data have been promoted as a means of improving service quality through increased accountability and transparency (Hermann & Provost, 2003). Performance data enable service providers, service users and funding bodies to monitor the performance of a given organisation relative to its peers on selected parameters. This motivates organisations to achieve higher performance and to strive for service provision that is of an acceptable standard (Shepherd *et al.*, 2010).

The collection, reporting and investigation of benchmarking data follow a recognised procedure (Box 18.1). In the initial stage, benchmarking partners identify what indicators

---

Box 18.1   A benchmarking process

1. Preparation, in which the following are determined:
   - what to benchmark
   - who or what to benchmark against
2. Comparisons, which may include the following activities:
   - data collection
   - data manipulation, construction of indicators, etc.
   - comparison of results with benchmarking partners
3. Investigation, that is, identification of practices and processes that result in superior performance
4. Implementation, in which best practices are adapted and/or adopted
5. Evaluation, where new practices are monitored to ensure continuous improvement and, if necessary the whole cycle is repeated

---

they wish to compare. Data are then collected on these indicators using the same data collection template to ensure consistency in the data collected. Services are then compared and activities leading to higher performance are investigated. These practices are then implemented in all services and the process is repeated.

Benchmarking in practice

Sam has been participating (with a number of colleagues) in a residential rehabilitation programme for the past 3 months. One component of the programme focuses on healthy living and weight control (please refer to Chapter 12 in this book). While all participants in the programme have lost weight since joining (average loss of 5.5 kg), you have no way of knowing if the weight loss achieved by the group is in keeping with best practice. You contact the manager of a similar programme in another region and a decision is made to share information on a number of performance indicators around weight (age of clients, diagnosis, weight on entry to programme, medication use, exercise programme, diet, etc.). The results indicate that clients in the comparison programme lost a total of 12.6 kg (more than double that of the clients in Sam's group).

A visit to the comparison programme is recommended at this stage to observe, first hand, how the different components of the programme operate. While visiting the programme, you learn that there is a greater emphasis on client education about diet and meal preparation. One major difference is that a dietician visits the programme twice a week to show clients how to cook low-fat meals and motivate them to participate in regular exercise. This strategy may have resulted in the superior weight loss in that programme. You source a dietician for your programme and 6 months later, another round of benchmarking is conducted to monitor the impact of having the dietician involved.

Thus, benchmarking is a continuous process of data collection, analysis and investigation so as to improve practice. In this scenario, there were only two services involved but the same approach can be used to evaluate the relative performance of many services at once.

The advantages of benchmarking can extend beyond simple data collection. Benchmarking encourages services to discuss programmes and how they are structured

---

Box 18.2   Advantages of benchmarking

- Assists in establishing systems of ongoing monitoring and evaluation
- Motivates services to implement change through peer pressure
- Provides opportunities for services to discuss optimal structures and procedures
- Identifies weaknesses in practice models and encourages implementation of remedial strategies
- Assists with securing data for accreditation and overall programme evaluation

---

and delivered. It can also improve cohesion between services and this places increased pressure on services that are performing less strongly to address potential reasons (Box 18.2).

Summary

Evaluation of programmes has often been neglected by services in the past. However, services and individual practitioners are accountable to clients and funders to deliver services that are engaging, accurately apply strategies that are known to work, and are effective in terms of client impacts and outcomes. Programme evaluation enables us to meet this duty and address issues that may be impeding optimal outcomes. Benchmarking enables services to help each other to solve problems with implementation and to meet objectives. Programme evaluation is not an added extra to be done if funding and time permit – it is a core responsibility we all have.

Resource

A valuable set of programme evaluation resources can be accessed through the Centers for Disease Control and Prevention (CDC) website at http://www.cdc.gov/eval/resources/index.htm.

References

Berg M, Meijerink Y, Gras M *et al.* (2005) Feasibility first: developing public performance indicators on patient safety and clinical effectiveness for Dutch hospitals. *Health Policy* **75**, 59–73.

Bullivant J (1994) *Benchmarking for Continuous Improvement in the Public Sector.* Longman: Harlow, Essex.

Donabedian A (1966) Evaluating the quality of medical care. *Milbank Memorial Fund Quarterly* **44**, 166–206.

Hermann R, Provost S (2003) Interpreting measurement data for quality improvement: standards, means, norms, and benchmarks. *Psychiatric Services* **54**, 655–7.

Meehan T, Stedman T, Neuendorf K, Francisco I, Neilson G (2007) Benchmarking Australia's mental health services: is it possible and useful? *Australian Health Review* **31**, 623–7.

Shepherd N, Meehan T, Davidson F, Stedman T (2010) Evaluation of benchmarking initiatives in extended treatment mental health services. *Australian Health Review* **34**, 1–6.

Stufflebeam D (1971) *Educational Evaluation and Decision Making*. Peackock: Itasca, Illinois.

Teague GB, Bond GR, Drake RE (1998) Program fidelity in assertive community treatment: development and use of a measure. *American Journal of Orthopsychiatry* **68**, 216–32.

Index

Manual of Psychosocial Rehabilitation, First Edition. Edited by Robert King, Chris Lloyd, Tom Meehan,
Frank P. Deane and David J. Kavanagh.
© 2012 Blackwell Publishing Ltd. Published 2012 by Blackwell Publishing Ltd.